special ~~£7.50~~

£3-75

~~43711~~
~~230 D1~~
115D2

Coping with Uncertainty

Policy and Politics in the National Health Service

SOCIAL POLICY RESEARCH MONOGRAPHS SERIES

Series Editor: **Dr. Hans Wirz,**
Department of Social Administration, University of Edinburgh, Scotland

1. Teamwork for Preventive Care
Nigel Bruce

2. Coping with Uncertainty: Policy and Politics in the National Health Service
David J. Hunter

Coping with Uncertainty

Policy and Politics in the National Health Service

David J. Hunter
Royal Institute of Public Administration, London, England

RESEARCH STUDIES PRESS
A DIVISION OF JOHN WILEY & SONS LTD
Chichester · New York · Brisbane · Toronto

RESEARCH STUDIES PRESS

Editorial Office:
8 Willian Way, Letchworth, Herts SG6 2HG, England

British Library Cataloguing in Publication Data:

Hunter, David J
Coping with uncertainty.
- (Social policy research monograph series).
1. Health services administration - Great Britain
- Decision making
2. Great Britain. National Health Service
I. Title II. Series
362.1 RA395.G6 80-41270

ISBN 0 471 27906 4

Printed in the United States of America

Most of the evidence suggests that real management work is characterised by variety, discontinuity and brevity. Managers work in power networks, armed with informal information and at high speed. Decision-making, one of the main planks of the rational/ scientific management idea, tends to be done through the seat of the pants, or off the top of the head, or in some other place, but rarely in an orderly, 'scientific' fashion.

Alistair Mant, The Rise and Fall of the British Manager, Macmillan, London, 1977, p.30.

Contents

Tables

Diagrams

Acknowledgements

The case material which forms the core of the book is based on research carried out between 1975 and 1977. The fieldwork involved numerous individuals in the two health boards selected for study, including members, officers and representatives of various professions. They tolerated my presence and inquiries with patience and good humour. I am most grateful to all of them for their co-operation and generous hospitality and to the ten other health boards which responded so readily to my questionnaire.

I am, of course, indebted to my two research supervisors, Susan Sinclair (Department of Social Administration, University of Edinburgh) and Charles Raab (Department of Politics, University of Edinburgh), for their guidance and support. I am grateful also to my two examiners, Professor Raymond Illsley (MRC Medical Sociology Unit, University of Aberdeen) and Michael Clarke (Deputy Director, Policy Planning Unit, Lothian Region), for their helpful suggestions and comments on the original thesis. I also wish to express my appreciation to those who provided opportunities to discuss my research at various stages of completion. In particular, thanks go to Drummond Hunter, Secretary, Scottish Health Service Planning Council; Rex Taylor, MRC Medical Sociology Unit, University of Aberdeen; Kenneth Boyd, Edinburgh Medical Group; Mike Porter, Department of General Practice, University of Edinburgh; and Alan Davis, University of Sydney, Australia. Needless to say, none of the above is responsible for any faults or errors in what follows.

I have also profited from my work on the NHS carried out at the Outer Circle Policy Unit which, thanks to the Unit's Director, James Cornford, has enabled me to pursue my interest at a time when the NHS is in a state of turbulence. This work has brought me into contact with many in the health field, both academics and practitioners, too numerous to mention here.

I reserve a special thanks to my wife, Mairi, who lived with the thesis for as long as I care to remember only to have the gap left by its completion filled by the preparation of this book. She has not only helped directly through the provision of essential support services and through checking the final typescript but, as ever, her encouragement and devotion have been indispensable.

I was supported during this project by a studentship from the Social Science Research Council.

Part of the material contained in Chapters 1, 3 and 6 first appeared in the following publications: Sociology of Health and Illness, 1, No 1, June 1979 (published by Routledge and Kegan Paul), and Appendix 2 in K M Boyd, ed., The Ethics of Resource Allocation in Health Care, Edinburgh, University Press, Edinburgh, 1979.

David J Hunter
London
February 1980

Foreword

Problems produce recipes for their solution. Whereas cooks can taste the results of recipes soon after their creation, and resolve never to try the recipe again, the costs and benefits of new formulae for making great bureaucracies work more smoothly, emerge slowly. When David Hunter began his study of decision-making in the NHS, structural reorganisation of the system, involving much upheaval, and some optimism, had barely been completed. It can never be undone and few people could contemplate with pleasure the thought of further change on that scale. The Royal Commission on the NHS decided that it was the best system we have and recommended nuts-and-bolts reform rather than structural solutions. A new consensus is emerging that structural change does not solve political problems and may not even have much effect on established professional behaviour. Dr Hunter's conclusions suggest that, instead of solving problems, massive structural change may obscure the pertinent issues, direct attention towards administrative and managerial technicalties and leave the sources of unease untouched and postponed for future political solution. The central problem is undoubtedly a political one, for it is concerned with how to shift resources from one use to another, from one group of service-providers to another and therefore from one client group to another. Priorities may be defined by national governments (or perhaps more accurately by government departments and their professional advisers) but, in organisations dominated by semi-autonomous professionals, the chain of implementation is long and subject to modification and distortion in every link. Evidence accumulates that, within broad limits, policy is made at the spending end through the innumerable daily acts of many practitioners. This does not signify incompetence or ill-will but the natural tendency of persons equipped with specific skills and with professionally-inculcated perspectives and definitions of health and disease to interpret their task accordingly. And since highly trained professionals must have wide powers of discretion in order to act effectively and with motivation, pressure and accommodation is a more appropriate strategy than enforcement.

The structural reorganisation of the NHS was accomplished with a minimum scientific sociological input. As Dr Hunter states it was based on a model of decision-making which assumed a set of clear, objective, technical precepts and rational linking of ends and means. Management criteria were consequently over-emphasised. The model which envisages the NHS as a loose organisation of separate groupings with different interests and objectives, and decision-making as a process of negotiation, was overlooked. I would perpetuate the same fallacy if I claimed that, had they been able to read Dr Hunter's report, all would have been different. It is, however, true that very few first-hand scientific accounts exist of the internal workings of the NHS. The number of medical sociologists and of students of social administration is small, and of these few have concerned themselves with the formulation and implementation of health policy. The major deficiency however has lain, not in numbers but in access, for Health Boards and even more so, the Health Departments, are relatively closed to the detailed, searching inquiry into intimate matters which Dr Hunter achieved. This book is valuable for its intrinsic method but also for being a very rare sociological glimpse into the inside. If structural change brings limited benefits and many costs, if enforcement is impracticable, we shall have to rely more heavily in future on similar studies to achieve that understanding of 'process' which is so important to the dynamics and outcome of policy implementation.

With hindsight, it is clear that the process of decision-making through which Development Funds came to be allocated could have achieved no other result than the fair-shares, balancing-out, 'a bit here and a bit there' outcome which Dr Hunter describes. Nor had we seen, from the inside, the multiple pressures and constraints upon those involved in the process. Perhaps most disturbing at a time when shifts in resources between committed professionals and their services are needed for adaptation to new definitions of health and of need, is the marginal contribution to policy-making and implementation of Health Board Members. I hope that the publication of Dr Hunter's work will stimulate more research, and some action, on such important issues.

Professor Raymond Illsley
Director MRC Medical Sociology Unit
Aberdeen

CHAPTER 1

Introduction

We know little about how public policy is formed in Britain. This study aims partially to remedy our ignorance by lifting a corner of the veil which conceals decision-making in the NHS. It describes the findings of a two year research project which involved observing a series of financial decisions undertaken in two Scottish health boards. The findings are interesting not only for what they reveal about operating practices in the NHS at local level, but also for their illumination of a theoretical approach that is of value in accounting for the actual mechanics of decision-making.

There are sound reasons for believing that it is both important and necessary to understand decision processes in a sphere of activity, like health care, that impinges on us all at some stage in our lives. Although it may seem remarkable that there is a dearth of studies describing what happens within field authorities comprising the NHS, an absence of case studies of how administrators, and others, go about their work is evident throughout the field of public administration in Britain (1). Books on public administration, as Ridley (2) has noted:

> 'embody little research into what actually goes on inside the administration ... The administration ... is the box in which inputs are actually translated into outputs ... The way the box is organised, its pattern of work and communication system, for

example, is bound to affect (the policy process').

Most work on public administration has been content merely to describe what institutions are, rather than what they do. Although valuable, studies of this kind make no attempt, often intentionally, to come to terms with the dynamics of decision-making and with the political realities involved. They centre on structural questions, such as the size of authorities and the distribution of powers within these authorities, rather than on questions of process and of the actual behaviour of people within formal structures.

A growing number of studies have attempted to correct this imbalance and, at the same time, overcome what Stanyer (3) refers to as 'the legalism and institutionalism' that have dominated studies of government and public authorities. Most of the new literature on the dynamics of decision-making, and on the political realities that are inseparable from decision processes, is concerned with local government and related services, in particular education (4). For instance, Stanyer's approach to understanding local government involves perceiving local authorities as individual miniature political systems in their own right, each with its own distinctive character. The policy-making and budgetary processes in local authorities are now receiving attention equal to their importance although there is scope for further work.

However, when it comes to the NHS there is less evidence of academic interest in organisational and/or political issues, particularly at a local level (5). This is partly a consequence of the direction taken by most research coming into the category of medical sociology. While considerable attention has been devoted to the professional/bureaucratic dilemma within health care systems (6), most medical sociology has been confined to definitions of disease and to studies of doctor/patient relationships (7), and organisational and political questions relating to the planning and delivery of services have been neglected. There is, then, a strong argument for shifting attention from decision-making in clinical settings to decision-making in administrative structures (8).

While valuable, studies of NHS policy-making on a national level (9) have served to emphasise the paucity of data about what goes on within local health authorities. Obviously, analyses from both central and local perspectives are necessary and ought to complement each other, but there are sound reasons for shifting the emphasis to the local arena and to what Kogan (10) terms 'the fine grain of social systems and what they have to do' since they are 'the sites of the real social action'. Surprising though it may seem, the reorganisation of the NHS in 1974 was carried through without any study of decision processes having been commissioned (11). In view of the major changes which were put in train, it surely a significant omission. It is not surprising, therefore, that Stanyer and Smith (12) are critical of administrative reform in Britain between 1966 and 1976.

> 'Neither the student of public administration nor the citizen ... can be satisfied with the present state of affairs. The processes of investigation, analysis and advice about the machinery of government do not justify the words used to commend them when, for instance, a Royal Commission is created. The cynical view is undoubtedly realistic; reform arises from political demands or political expediency, and the language of rational discovery is a facade'.

As if to reinforce this damning indictment of the (mis) management of institutional reform in Britain, at the time of writing it is possible that the government may repeat the events leading to the upheaval in 1974 if it proceeds with its proposals for restructuring the Service in the wake of the report of the Royal Commission on the NHS which expressed misgivings about the cumbersome structure to emerge from reorganisation (13).

If the primary aim of government policy in the NHS is to increase the rationality of decision-making (and this was a key theme running through the 1974 reforms), a thorough appreciation of existing procedures would appear to be an essential prerequisite. Relevant knowledge on the realities of decision-making is necessary and indeed indispensable, since sensible reforms (one can argue about what these might be) must depend on knowledge of the world as it is, just as much as on knowledge of the world as it ought to be. In the case of the NHS, until a more adequate description is developed of what actually happens in health authorities, where policy is largely formulated and implemented, proposals for reform will continue to be based upon inadequate understanding. This does not augur well for their success.

There is already substantial evidence to show that central government policy in health care, as manifested in the NHS, has not been notable for its success (14). Not only have stubborn regional imbalances remained during the 30 odd years since the NHS was created, but priorities between care groups have not been easy to alter. The second concern which prompted the present study was puzzlement at the persistence of resource imbalances as between different sectors of health care, as between different health authorities and particularly within health authorities, and a desire to discover what influences and constraints operated upon decision-makers to account for these inequities. The existence of these imbalances was another reason for reorganising the NHS (15). Research to date in this area has not investigated, in any depth, decision-makers' own perceptions of the issues involved and the difficulties which arise from their operating environment (16). For example, do the imbalances which exist between services arise from the power relations within health authorities? Do they emanate from a desire not to disturb vested interests? Or do they exist as a result of the uncertainty of the environment: decision-makers simply do not know what to do or how to do it? Heclo (17) has written: 'social policy-making is about puzzlement as well as power; it entails both knowing and deciding'. It may be that in an uncertain environment, administrators strive for stability and order, instead of promoting innovation, and that this accounts for the overwhelming tendency to maintain the <u>status quo</u>. Schon (18) has termed this reaction 'dynamic conservatism' (i.e. people 'fight like mad to stay where they are'). It is not simply a question of medical politics dictating what decisions emerge, although undeniably such activity is of relevance. Possibly, the process is more subtle than crude power politics, for the reasons Heclo states. The NHS decision-making environment is, or can be, highly uncertain. Preventive care illustrates this. No one is quite sure what preventive care means or involves in the way of specific policies and services. Is a health education programme worth initiating? Should mass screening programmes be started? How does one measure the return on investment? The entire preventive field is riddled with such questions. Answers may be forthcoming one day, but meantime administrators and others are involved in what might be termed 'cautious groping'.

In discussing the imbalances in service provision that occur within health authorities, it quickly becomes apparent that decision-making in the NHS is far more decentralised than might be supposed or is often argued. For example, Enoch Powell (19), when Minister of Health, maintained that the NHS was over-centralised, whereas Richard Crossman (20), when Secretary of State for Social Services, believed quite vehemently that the centre lacked sufficient control over health authorities. He describes how difficult it was to shift resources from acute services, to those in the 'Cinderella' sectors of health care. Klein (21) shares Crossman's views. The NHS is run by the centre on a loose rein and is, in fact, a good example of decentralised decision-making (22). This is not to say that the centre never interfers authoritatively with health authorities but it rarely does so, or its attempts to do so tend to be distorted or suborned. Reorganisation of the NHS was, in large part, an attempt to improve the centre's ability to decide overall priorities and thereby influence the day-to-day decisions taken by the field authorities. But health authorities continue to possess a large measure of administrative influence over the services they provide. There is a distinction between the controls central government has over health authorities, and their actual operation. What needs to be recognised is the political dimension,

'... complex interactions take place within a system of administrative politics ...' (23). Just as local authorities should be seen as political entities, with shifting routines and allegiances, so should health authorities be seen as political arenas with shifting routines and allegiances.

STUDY AIMS

For present purposes, policy-making may be regarded as synonymous with the term decision-making, since the study concerns itself with decisions involving more strategic levels of choice than is the case with simple routine decision-making, which has no direct policy impact (24). The decision-making activities which form the empirical core of the study are not examples of policy-making directed towards the improvement of, say, geriatric services or acute services as functional groupings, i.e. macro-policy-making. As between routine decision-making at one extreme and macro-policy-making at the other, the decision processes with which the research is concerned, fall within the category of middle-range decision-making. The outcomes of middle-range decision-making at health board level can have an impact on broader, more strategic policy-making activity. Indeed, middle-range decision-making is often a substitute for macro-policy-making, which aims at a more synoptic approach and one that decision-makers find difficulty in adopting.

Nearly all policies involve spending and, therefore, policy-making and budgeting (i.e. the process of allocating financial resources to particular ends) are invariably inseparable. The case study is concerned with a particular area of the budgetary process in health authorities, and seeks answers to questions like the following: how are scarce resources allocated? Who is involved in these decisions? How are choices made between competing demands? Is there a hierarchy of power or influence? What information is used in the discussions surrounding the decision-making process? In short, it is the intention of the case study to go some way towards eliminating the ignorance identified earlier, by untangling the processes involved in reaching certain types of resource-allocation decisions in the NHS. It proceeds by identifying the actors, the constraints, the coping strategies and the political forces which help to shape decisions.*

The greater part of the funds allocated to each health board is already earmarked for existing commitments. Although theoretically these funds could be put to different uses, in practice they are not. The budgets remain fixed. In the jargon, there are no 'zero-base reviews'. The case study focuses upon the 'new' money which a health board receives annually from the Scottish Office for developing the Service. Development Funds (DF) enable a health board to develop new services, improve existing ones, or to change direction as a result of a new emphasis having been placed on certain services. It is in connection with the allocation of these funds that one may best observe the processes which are involved in deciding how the Service is to be developed. Particularly interesting are the sorts of calculations and tactics that are deployed in discussions concerning the allocation of DF. In short, whatever the significance of the <u>substance</u> of any decision, it is the <u>process</u> of decision-making which is of primary concern.

The vantage point offered by a concentration on budgeting decisions provides a useful, and much-neglected, perspective from which to analyse the making of policy in health care. Wildavsky (25) claims that the task of allocating money can explain, or help to explain, how people at various levels in an organisation co-operate, bargain and negotiate. The struggle for money is a pervasive and informative operation about what goes on in an organisation.

---

* Although the case study was carried out in Scotland whose health service differs in some important respects from health services elsewhere in the UK (see Chapter 2), the processes observed, and the findings to emerge, have a much wider relevance. What happens in Scotland appears, on the strength of other similar research, to parallel closely what happens in England. Less is known about Wales and Northern Ireland although it is unlikely that they would differ greatly, especially Wales.

Since funds are limited and have to be divided in one way or another, the budget becomes a mechanism for making choices among alternative expenditures. If politics is regarded as the conflict (either overt or covert) over whose preferences shall prevail in the determination of policy, then the budget records the outcome of this struggle. 'Human nature is never more evident than when men are struggling to gain a larger share of the funds or to apportion what they have among myriad claimants ... The budget lies at the heart of the political process' (26). A study of resource-allocation decisions can indicate what pressures make for policy change or for policy maintenance (27), and whence these originate.

The central actors in the decision process observed can be grouped into three categories which collectively form a policy triad: (a) Health Board - governing body; (b) Officers - area, district and sector; (c) Advisory Groups - professional and consumer. The interactions among these groups, and within them, and the resources available to each, are explored in subsequent chapters. Anticipating what lies ahead, the main findings to emerge from the study may be noted in outline here. The case study, as mentioned, set out to understand more fully than hitherto the mechanics of development fund allocations and the involvement of the policy triad in these. The study revealed, first, a series of constraints on decision-makers, such as time and the availability of information, and, secondly, a range of tactics and coping strategies which were deployed to circumvent or manage these, and other, anomalies. The study also discovered that tensions arising from the operation of the management structure introduced when the NHS was reorganised in 1974 created additional difficulties for those entrusted with the task of allocating funds (28). The findings are particularly revealing in the context of the 1974 reforms which were designed to achieve a more effective and efficient use of resources. These findings are important too at a time when resources for health services are scarce and when further structural reform is firmly on the political agenda.

PLAN OF BOOK

Chapter 2 provides essential background for the case study and its narrow focus on development fund allocations in two health boards. The uniqueness of the NHS as a large and complex organisation is briefly noted and the events surrounding the re-organisation of the NHS are reviewed, with particular attention being paid to those features that have a direct bearing on the specific focus of the case study. The budgeting arrangements in the NHS, as these operate in Scotland, are also described.

In Chapter 3, the theoretical and methodological foundations of the case study are laid and there is a discussion of the merits and/or demerits of the analytical approaches of the rationalists on the one hand and the incrementalists on the other. These theories, and their derivatives, are reviewed for their potential in helping to elucidate the allocation process described in the case study from the varied perspectives of the participants in that process.

The next three chapters form the empirical core of the research. Chapters 4 and 5 focus on the determination of policy through the allocation of development funds over a two year period. By giving detailed accounts of what actually happened, the narrative shows the interrelationships and manoeuvrings between the groups of decision actors comprising the policy triad. In Chapter 6 an attempt is made to stand back from the detailed descriptive accounts and present an analysis of the allocation process as well as an explanation of how decision actors come to terms with their environment.

Finally, Chapter 7 draws some conclusions from the case study in regard to the activities of health boards, officers and professionals, in regard to decision-making and planning in such an environment and in regard to current moves to alter the structural shape of the NHS. The relevance of decision-making theory in contributing to a better understanding of how the decisions described in the case study emerged is also considered. Even if broad generalisations are not realistically possible, drawn as they would have to be from only one case study, it is hoped that the study will provide some valuable insights into the operation of the NHS at health authority level. If it contributes to a deeper understanding of that process, its purpose will have been more than adequately served.

CHAPTER 2

The National Health Service: An Overview

The NHS is a distinctive type of formal organisation which deviates somewhat from the Weberian model of bureaucracy (1). What is unique about it is that it is a split organisation, with a bureaucratic component and a professional component (2). It is the nature of this split organisation which underlies many of the management problems and tensions in the NHS, before and since reorganisation, and which hinders the bringing about of a more equitable use of resources between different sectors of health care (3).

The type of organisation found in the NHS, and the distribution of power and authority within it, is deeply affected by the doctor's special relationship to his patients (i.e. the concept of clinical autonomy, arising directly out of the nature of the doctor-patient relationship, which has been enshrined in all official reports concerned with the organisation of the NHS). There are other so-called 'professional' groups in the NHS, notably nurses, but the medical profession has a unique authority (4). Rowbottom (5) has written:

> 'the position of doctors ... presents a fascinating, and possibly unique, situation to any student of organisation. Never have so many highly influential figures been found in such an equivocal position - neither wholly of, nor wholly divorced from, the organisation which they effectively dominate'.

What constitutes a profession will not be the subject of lengthy discussion here. Suffice it to say that the study of professions to date has, with one or two notable exceptions, tended to accept unquestioningly professionals' own definitions of themselves (6). There have been few attempts to understand professional occupations in terms of their resources of power and the ways in which they use them. The resources of power of any profession depend largely upon the esoteric character of its knowledge or expertise, as this affects the degree of autonomy and influence which a profession possesses. Knowledge itself does not give special power, but rather the fact of organised occupations which have exclusive access to such knowledge. It is in this sense that the professions should be viewed as inseparable from political processes. Knowledge and skill are claimed by a group to advance its interests. Claims to such expertise are thus unlikely to remain neutrally descriptive. They function as professional ideologies which can either be a function of crude self-interest, or they can be seen as natural outcomes of a deep commitment to the value of the work a profession does (7). This orientation helps to explain why each profession tends to perceive the world in terms of its own conception of problems and solutions, and why in the political arena each tries to argue for more resources as a way of advancing the general good. This latter point emerges strongly in the case study presented in later chapters.

A feature of the NHS is the interaction and interplay between the deliverers of health care (primarily the medical profession, but other occupations are also involved), the administrators (lay and professional) who control the resources and who are responsible for the day-to-day running of the Service, and the health board (the governing body which is largely composed of lay members). The relationship between the medical profession and administrators in the management of the NHS is of particular interest, since the aims and objectives of each group are generally rather different: doctors insist upon complete clinical freedom to treat every patient in the manner that they individually see to be in the patient's best interests, and they see themselves as being accountable only to the patients whom they serve and to their own conscience; administrators, on the other hand, are concerned with the operation of the NHS as a whole, rather than with the specific needs of individual patients, and they see their purpose as one of achieving a more economic, efficient and effective use of limited resources. The relationship between these two groups is crucial in the operation of the NHS, and may be expected to become even more significant during a prolonged period of nil growth.

Four aspects of the medical profession's influence on the NHS deserve consideration. These are not dealt with at any length in the case study, but form an essential part of the background to it. They are: (a) the medical profession and clinical autonomy; (b) the authority of the medical profession in relation to other professions; (c) the extent to which one medical profession can be said still to exist; and (d) the relationship of the medical profession(s) to the management of health services.

Under (a), much of the medical profession's influence is derived from the rather nebulous concept of clinical autonomy. Administrators have no right to direct in the area of care and treatment, they can only discuss and persuade. 'Doctors to date have for the most part been given blank cheques to make whatever demands upon the system that they individually see fit' (8). It is at this interface, where the immovable object of clinical autonomy meets the force of resource constraints, that the most interesting characteristics of decision-making in the NHS may be observed. Here, the groups of decision actors which form the policy triad (health board members, officers and advisory bodies) converge to negotiate, persuade and bargain.

Under (b), the authority of the medical profession in relation to other health care occupations is a subject of increasing importance. For instance, do such relationships strengthen the medical profession's autonomy, or do they weaken it by acting as constraints upon it? Is the hegemony of the medical profession at an end? These questions are considered below.

Under (c), in addition to inter-professional

relationships, intra-professional rivalries are now a major feature of the medical profession and of medical politics generally. It is no longer accurate to speak of one medical profession; rather there are many, as is described below.

Under (d), the fourth aspect of influence of the medical profession(s) is in its (their) relationship to the management of the Service and to those 'lay' elements within management (i.e. 'lay' in the sense of not containing a medical component; for example, administration and finance). There are two main ways in which doctors, and some other groups of employees, like nurses, may participate in the management structure of the NHS. One is as individuals interacting with the governing body so as to affect policy-formation by individual advice, persuasion and pressure (medical administrators function in this way, as do Community Medicine Specialists). The other is through the formation of groups, which agree common views and policies and then, again by advice, persuasion and pressure, try to influence policy-formation with elected representatives acting as their spokesmen. This second channel is of prime importance in medical organisation. One result of the reorganisation of the NHS has been a plethora of advisory committees at most levels of the management hierarchy. In a series of official reports (9) the medical profession has been exhorted to participate fully in the management of the NHS.

However, while the medical profession may possess the potential to exert considerable influence over matters, such as resource-allocation decisions, there are constraints operating to counteract this. These are important, since they relate to the crucial matter of 'medical dominance' in priority-setting. There are three clearly identifiable constraints. While some documentation of them exists, confirmation of their importance was provided by the case study.

First, the medical profession itself acts as a constraint. It is no longer as homogeneous as it was several decades ago, before the upsurge of medicine and medical technology. Developments in medicine, amounting to a scientific revolution in health, have resulted in the emergence of many new specialties, including neurosurgery, cardiac surgery, radiology, psychiatry and so on. Such a proliferation has had the effect of weakening the unity of the profession as a whole, which may lead to fragmentation, divergences of opinion between different specialties being a clear possibility. Illness trends have had a similar effect. Concern with prevention and a shift from policies aimed at curing to those aimed at caring have weakened the status and unity of the medical profession. Other, more longstanding, divisions are apparent too, between consultants and junior doctors, and between hospital doctors and general practitioners. Bevan capitalised on some of these intra-professional rivalries in order to establish the NHS in 1948 (10).

Second, in keeping with changing techniques and disease patterns, doctors are becoming more and more dependent on the services provided by a host of paramedical occupations, like nurses who, although a 'cut above' the rest in the NHS hierarchy, have not quite attained professional status, laboratory technicians, radiographers, physiotherapists, dieticians etc. These groups act as constraints on the medical profession's hegemony because although in the past they were subservient to doctors, the latter now have to consider the views of these groups and accommodate them. Armstrong (11) notes a gradual decline in strength of the medical hegemony over the last 25 years and argues that an increasing division of medical labour represents a challenge to medical dominance. Disputes in recent years in the NHS over pay and private practice have involved many of these paramedical and ancillary groups and have served to illustrate the interrelatedness of modern health care, and the indispensability of the skills and services they provide. Moreover, the reorganised NHS has provided the paramedical occupations with channels of influence denied them before 1974. Their influence on decision-making may be expected to grow.

A third, and final, constraint is constituted by the failure of the medical profession to become properly involved in the management of the NHS. There is some evidence to suggest that doctors regard committee work as a chore and many, if not most of them, try to avoid it or are ill-prepared for it. Reorganisation has increased the management tasks of clinicians; many, or most, are on some kind of committee. In evidence to the Royal Commission on the NHS, a team of management consultants from McKinsey and Company (12) suggest that 'the consultative machinery is too cumbersome and represents over-insurance by the professions involved'. The authors argue that unnecessary consultation is time consuming. 'In some areas, as many as one doctor in three is a member of some committee or team, taking up substantial amounts of his time' (13). There is, however, an ambivalence in attitudes expressed by doctors. They want to be involved in management, and yet do not want to sacrifice valuable clinical time to the successful performance of a management role. In the longer term, they do not wish to compromise their clinical independence by assuming management functions. Yet, at the same time, securing a share of resources and determining priorities can only be done through involvement in management activities.

Apart from this ambivalence over management, and the existence of genuine constraints such as lack of time, it has been argued that clinicians, by virtue of their medical ideology, find extreme difficulty in functioning effectively as a corporate group (14). Reference has already been made to the concept of clinical autonomy and the ideological orientation of clinicians towards 'individualism'. Medical values militate against the formation of true collective action. This suggests, therefore, that whereas _individually_ doctors have (or had) power, _collectively_ they risk losing it. Prior to the 'Cogwheel' divisional system (15) and reorganisation, doctors wielded considerable influence as individuals. Since these events, doctors have been expected to operate collectively as members of teams and groups, and to reach a consensus on the issues before them. In short, doctors are now asked to give up individual power in order to achieve a collective say. It will not be easy for them to do this, especially when the end result of these changes _may_ be a diminution of the medical profession's influence as a corporate whole, although within the profession certain specialties may fare better than others.

The medical profession is by no means the only important group in the NHS, despite the fact that its influence does permeate (whether negatively or positively), the entire decision-making process. The operations of health boards and the relationships between members and officers remain obscure, since little is known about them. For example, what exactly does a health board do? What is its purpose? Is it necessary? Is a board anything other than a 'rubber-stamping' agency for decisions already effectively taken by the officers? Relationships among officers themselves at area, district and sector levels also remain mysteries, as do the ways in which they operate and their impact on decision processes. Finally, another set of relationships that is important in the functioning of the NHS, is that between the central department responsible for health and its agents, the field authorities, below. All these factors and relationships emerge at various points in the case study.

THE REORGANISED NHS IN SCOTLAND

The NHS in Scotland stands as an independently constituted Service, although much of its general plan is identical with that of the Service in England and Wales. It was established for the same needs and aims, and it is associated with a body of social legislation common to the United Kingdom. There are also certain matters, especially in the spheres of financial provision, parliamentary control, and in the regulation of professional conditions of service in which the two Services must act in common. However, the Scottish Health Service, while sharing many of the features of the English Health Service, is not a mere variant on the English model. Apart from obvious differences in the scale of operations between the two countries and differences in medical traditions (16), for present purposes the variations that are of interest are those that lie in the area of administration and policy. While there are significant differences in institutional arrangements, departures in policy have been more subtle.

Reorganisation of the NHS in Scotland occurred at the same time as the reorganisation of the Health Service in England and Wales, although the Scottish Act was passed by Parliament one year before the

English Act. Events moved more swiftly in Scotland because only one Green Paper was published prior to a white paper as opposed to two in England plus a consultative document. Reorganisation was deemed necessary for five main reasons, all interrelated. These applied more or less equally to England, Wales and Scotland.

The major obstacle posed by the former tripartite structure (see Diagram 1), was a lack of co-ordination and co-operation between the three separate parts of the NHS. This denied any continuity between primary care, hospital care and community care since these functions were organised under separate authorities. Some patients, to their detriment, fell between these somewhat arbitrary administrative boundaries. The 'frontier' problems became so acute that integration of the administrative structure was thought to be essential for a more comprehensive approach to health care. Second, the tripartite structure impeded effective planning across services and contributed to serious imbalances in priority setting and resource allocation. Planning was piecemeal, and no overall view of the Service was possible. Third, because costs were rising so steeply the need to use existing resources as effectively as possible was of paramount importance to national policy-makers. The NHS could not continue to devour an ever increasing proportion of a diminishing GNP (17). A unified NHS, it was believed, could lead to a better use of resources by switching the emphasis from acute hospital services to community services and long-stay care. Fourth, there was a view held by administrators, and by some doctors, that local authorities were slack in providing adequate community care services. It was alleged that since such services were not vote-catchers, they did not receive the priority that they ought to have had. Lack of co-ordination in service provision between the two sets of authorities resulted in patients being kept in hospital who ought not to have been there. Klein (18) has pointed out that many doctors in acute specialties favoured some form of re-organisation in the hope that their acute beds would cease to be clogged with patients who really ought to be treated in the community. Finally, politicians and civil servants saw reorganisation as an opportunity to challenge the exclusiveness of the medical profession in deciding what, and how, services should be provided and to whom. Attempts by various governments prior to reorganisation to redirect resources from acute services to the most vulnerable sectors within the NHS were not notable for their success. The extent to which reorganisation has been successful in meeting these five criticisms of the former structure is considered in the final chapter, in the light of the case study findings.

DIAGRAM 1 NATIONAL HEALTH SERVICE (SCOTLAND) 1948-1974

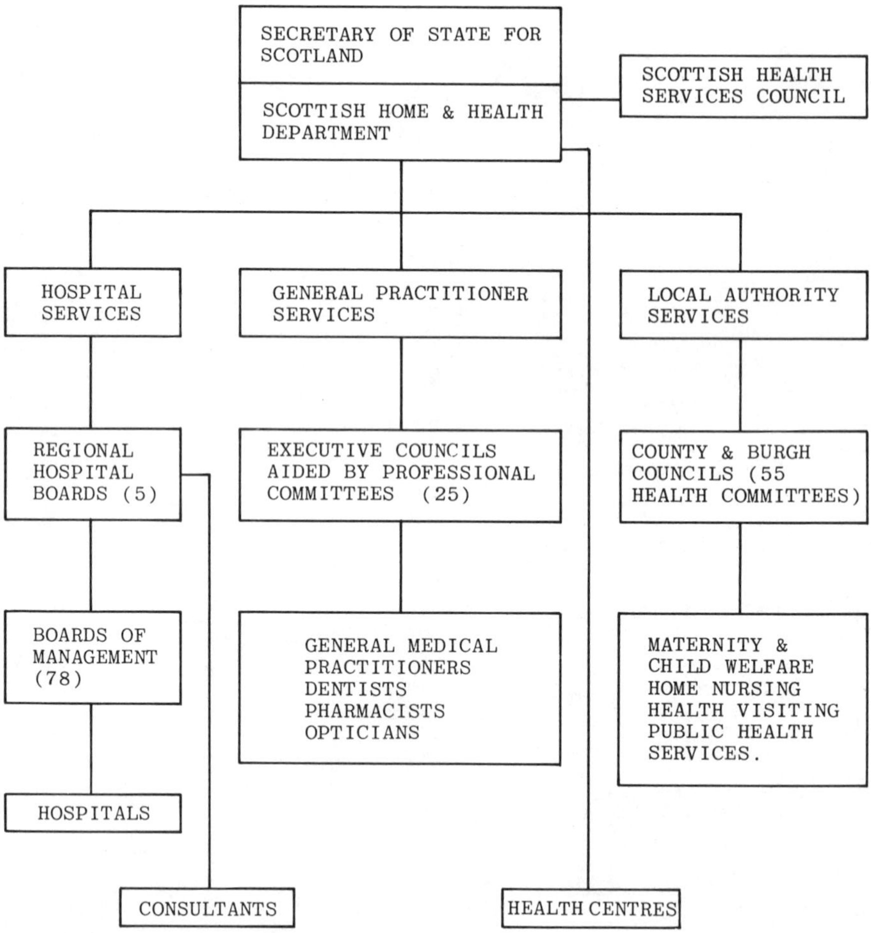

(a) The Structure

Ultimate responsibility for the administration of the health service in Scotland (see Diagram 2), rests with the Secretary of State for Scotland acting through the Scottish Office and, specifically, the Scottish Home and Health Department (SHHD). The Secretary of State is a member of the Cabinet, and is answerable to Parliament for his actions. Most day-to-day health matters are the responsibility of a junior Minister in the Scottish Office.

The main operational agencies of the Scottish Health Service are the fifteen health boards, ten of which have been divided into districts for management purposes. Below district level is a third layer of management, sectors, based either on a large individual hospital (or unit) or groups of smaller units, comprising hospitals and clinics together with community services. As in the case of most areas, the principle of coterminosity has been enshrined and, where possible, district boundaries have been drawn to coincide with one or more of the local government districts.

In terms of population, there is considerable variation among health boards. The largest board has a population of over 1 million, while the smallest has a population of 17,500. A cluster of boards comes within the population range 300,000 to 450,000, and the two boards featured in the case study have been selected from this group. The disparities between the remaining boards are too great to group conveniently. Membership of health boards also varies, with the largest boards having 22 members and the smallest having 14 members. In total there are 276 members, drawn from a wide range of interests, including industry, finance, commerce, farming, trade unions, universities, local government and health care professions. All, including the chairmen, are appointed by the Secretary of State for a term of four years which is renewable. According to one official document:

> 'Members are appointed for the contribution which they can make as individuals and, while they will be able to bring with them knowledge and experience from other spheres such as local government or

DIAGRAM 2 NATIONAL HEALTH SERVICE REORGANISATION SCOTLAND 1974

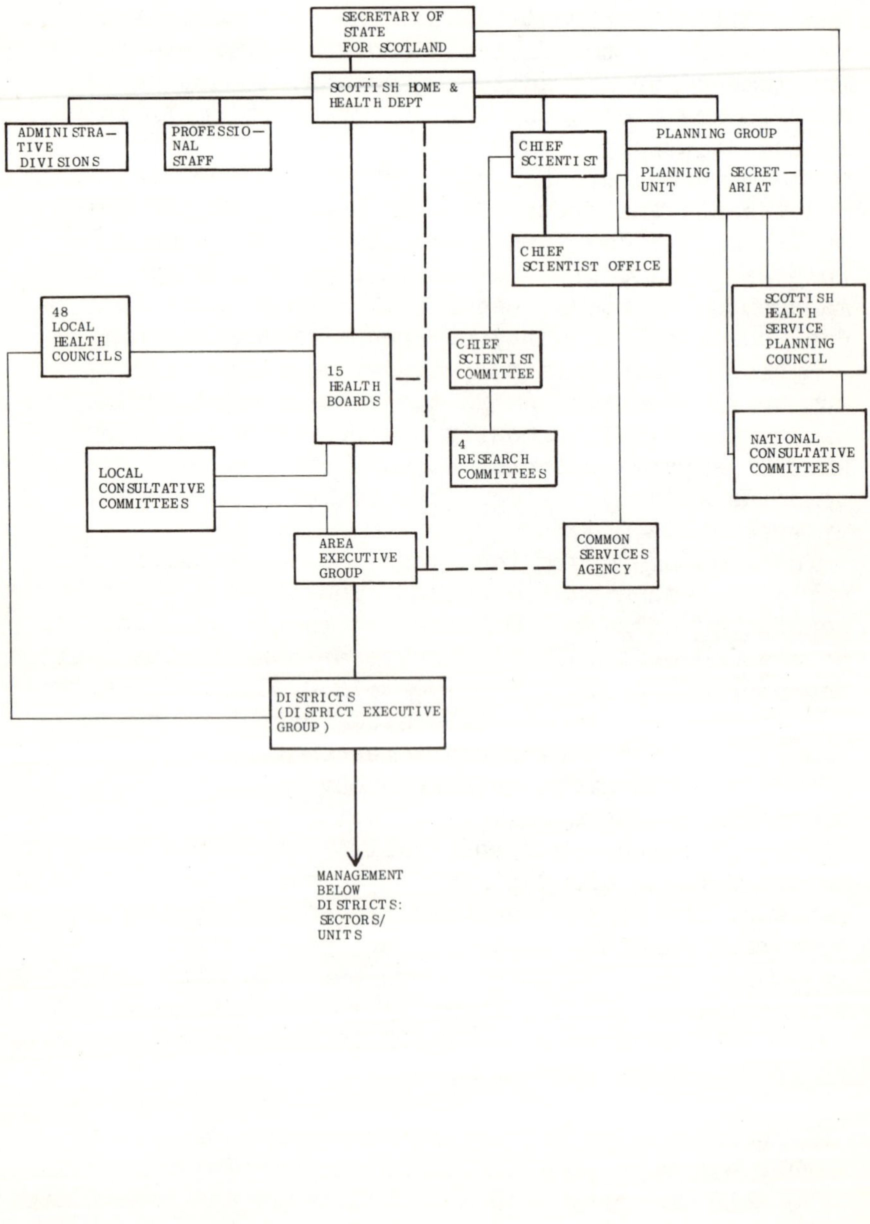

service within health establishments, it must be clear that they in no sense represent the interests by which they were nominated' (19).

This means that management and representation must be separate functions in order to avoid confusion between the two. It marks a departure from pre-reorganisation practice and has meant that the function of representing the public's interest in health care is now vested in separate Local Health Councils of which there are 48. However, the health board member's role has become complicated in that subsequent changes in the composition of boards, aimed at quelling growing criticism of the undemocratic nature of appointments, have led to an interweaving of representational and managerial elements (20). The result is that about one quarter of the membership on each board are local government nominees, two or three are trade union nominees, five have been nominated by the health care professions, one or two by universities and the balance, ranging from four to seven, have been nominated by other bodies. However, members are still expected to operate as individuals, not as representatives.

Health boards, when established in 1974, were responsible for deciding on how many, if any, districts would be needed in their respective areas. Factors which influenced the division of an area into districts included density of population, lines of communication, the organisation of existing health services, and the boundaries of local government districts (21). Ideally, 'the population comprised in a district should have a community of interest and a social coherence' (22). The subdivisions of districts, as mentioned, are called sectors and exist for (a) the management of institutions (i.e. hospitals, health centres, clinics); (b) the management of particular professional groups such as nurses; and (c) inter-professional co-operation in programmes directed to the care of specific groups of patients or people generally (23). Sector administration has been referred to as 'the neglected aspect of the management arrangements for the reorganised NHS' (24). This has occurred because the career structure of the administrator has become heavily weighted in favour of the higher management function at district and at area level.

(b) New Influences on Decision-making

Reorganisation of the NHS, in Scotland but especially elsewhere in the UK, has largely been about improved decision-making through the adoption of a particular managerial style, namely, one in which officers exercise substantial executive responsibility on behalf of their boards in the interests of the boards and their services. In this way it is hoped 'to make the most efficient use of resources' and to 'give effect as far as possible to the rational priorities of the community as a whole' (25).

Executive management at area and district levels is vested in the medical, nursing, administrative and financial officers who collectively form area and district executive groups which are corporate authorities, that is, they operate on a consensus basis, and on matters coming before them for decision they must reach unanimity. The purpose of an executive group at area level is to leave the board free to deal with 'major policy, strategic planning decisions, the broad allocation of resources and matters of substantial interest to the community' (26). District executive groups (DEGs) are responsible for the administration of integrated primary care, hospital services and community services within a specified boundary. Although accountable to area executive groups (AEGs), the intention is that DEGs should have a considerable degree of delegation. In England, the district is considered to be of great importance to the planning system operating there. The DHSS's planning guide (27) claims that:

> 'since most health services are delivered on a District basis, and most budgets are allocated within Districts, it is the District plan which will be the basic building block for the entire NHS annual planning system ... District plans will provide the basis for all annual planning in the NHS'.

In Scotland there is no planning system as such for

the NHS (see below) which may account for the different position occupied by the district in the management arrangements. The whole emphasis is different in Scotland, where health services are principally planned on an area basis. In the final analysis they are also managed on an area basis, with members of the DEGs being at all times the subordinates of their area counterparts. As one administrator commented in the interviews, control over the districts is 'much closer now than it ever was over Boards of Management.* There is not so much independence or detachment'. This changed relationship has been a source of friction (28) and it is explored in more detail in the case study. It is perhaps significant, in view of the different status of the district tier, that in England there is no line management relationship between district and area officers.

The officers comprising area and district executive groups have a dual role to perform in the new management structure. Each has his/her individual responsibilities as an officer. But, having become a member of an executive group, he/she also assumes responsibilities of a broader nature relating to the Service as a whole. Some of the problems associated with this dual role can be revealed more clearly if the operation of accountability in the structure is examined. It has two aspects. First, there is the accountability of individuals - of the district officer to his area counterpart, and of the area officer to the board; second, there is the accountability of groups - the DEG to the AEG, and the AEG to the board. There are difficulties in the accountability of individuals at district level to their superior at area level. For instance, the district officer cannot be a member of the area officer's immediate team because he is in a different kind of relationship. He is, in the first place, not just an assistant to the area officer, but a chief officer with his own set of responsibilities; second, he is

* Boards of Management were replaced in 1974. The nearest equivalent are districts. BoMs were accountable to 5 Regional Hospital Boards.

not near the area officer (in most cases) but is geographically separate; and third, his responsibilities are too weighty to be capable of daily adjustment with a 'superior'.

Greater problems arise over the operation of accountability between executive groups. In the previous two-tier system, Boards of Management (BoMs) were established as agents of Regional Hospital Boards (RHBs) and were responsible to RHBs for the management of hospitals. Immediate executive responsibility for the running of an individual hospital, or a group of hospitals, rested with the BoM while the RHB's main concern was to facilitate the efficient administration of the group by advisory function rather than by executive action. The Farquharson-Lang (29) committee, which examined administrative practices in hospital boards, reported the relationship in these terms: 'the functions of the two categories of Boards are therefore complementary'; the BoM exists 'to adjust the general administration of the hospital service to local conditions'. In practice this was a subtle, ambivalent, almost woolly, kind of relationship, since both authorities were boards of lay members possessing statutory powers. The new arrangements bear no resemblance to this structure. By comparison, relations between executive groups are stark and unambiguous.

The official circular (30) on these issues offers some guidance on the principles which apply to the delegation of powers to districts. It states that district management should be responsible to the executive of the board for providing the accepted level of service within an approved budget. Control over the district executive should be exercised by means of approved plans and financial budgets. 'The district executive should not normally refer to the AEG those decisions which it takes within its approved budget and in accordance with area policy', i.e. decisions which do not involve a change in area policy, a major change in the allocation of resources, or a major change in the services provided. This outline of the factors affecting relations between areas and districts begs several questions - for instance, how is the 'accepted' level of service determined? What is meant by 'approved plans'? When does a change in the allocation of resources become a major change? As implied above, where there are statutory authorities at both levels (i.e. pre-1974 NHS) the lines of responsibilities can be blurred at the edges, but in the present structure the relationships, for purposes of accountability, need to be clear-cut. Moving towards the correct balance is a matter which has occupied boards for a considerable time and some authorities, including the two observed in the case study, have questioned the necessity of districts in their particular areas. These structural and organisational issues inevitably have an influence on decision-making activities within health boards, even if it is not as profound as critics of the structure allege.

The importance of the executive group concept should not be underestimated. It has resulted in significant changes in the way in which the health service is administered in each area and, in particular, in the role now played by board members in decision-making. The requirement that executive groups at area and district levels must operate as consensus teams has, to some extent, formalised what was already happening in some authorities informally in the previous structure. However, it carries the process far beyond what went before. Prior to reorganisation, chief officers meeting as a group had no formal authority <u>as a group</u>. Decisions which required formal authority greater than that possessed by an individual officer, had to be taken by the board. Under existing arrangements, however, the executive group is not just a number of officers putting collective advice to the board. The executive group itself is vested with a collective authority to take decisions. On the one hand, officers formulate advice to the board on questions of policy, but, on the other, they themselves now take decisions, and on quite important matters. In addition, the executive group concept has enhanced the status of the nurse and treasurer in health service management. They are now equal members of the executive group, alongside the doctor and administrator.

The executive group concept is fundamental to the successful functioning of local health authorities.

An alternative approach to managing services at this level would have been to create two tiers of statutory authorities - area boards and district committees - and to provide each of them with sets of chief officers, without any reference to executive groups. In that event, the health service would have had the kind of pattern with which it was familiar prior to 1974 where each officer would have had a set of delegated powers and where there would have been no delegation to them as a group. Decisions which were important, either because of their magnitude or because they impinged on the interests of more than one chief officer, would have been referred to the board or committee, and all chief officers would have had an opportunity to tender advice as to the action which should be taken. Again, as in the past, it could happen that the chief officers might have previously discussed the matter and had been able to agree on the advice which they should jointly put to the board. Or it could happen that they had not met, or had met and not been able to agree, with the result that separate bits of advice would be offered to the board. The point to emphasise in all this is, that because the item of business would have been considered by the board, it would have been dealt with in a situation in which all aspects could be brought together and conflicting interests reconciled. The former boards and committees not only took decisions but exercised, by their very existence, this powerful co-ordinating influence.

In the new structure, there are three decision-taking and co-ordinating bodies - the board itself, the AEG and the DEG - but two of these bodies are composed entirely of officers. The dual role that officers now have is a combination of an officer role with a role analogous to that of a member, and, in its capacity to take decisions, the executive group of chief officers may be compared with an executive committee of board members. It should be stressed, however, that the decisions taken by executive groups fall within areas on which broad policy has been decided by the full board (e.g. a shift of emphasis towards geriatric care and away from acute services). Moreover, board members are fully entitled to question officers about decisions taken by executive groups. A further safeguard incorporated in the management arrangements is that the executive group can only take a decision if there is unanimous agreement. It is a consensus group and once a collective decision is taken each officer is committed to it. If an officer disagrees with other members of the group the matter has to be referred upwards for decision - to the board from the AEG, and to the AEG from the DEG.

Notwithstanding these checks and balances, there have been quite substantial changes in the operations of officers and board members, the result of which is that a great deal of decision-making lies not with board members, as it did prior to 1974, but with officers at area and district levels. The management style adopted has led to the creation of a system in which officers carrying major responsibilities are supervised by boards, instead of a system in which the concept is of boards assisted by officers. The arrangement is a reversal of roles for board members and officers (31). The executive groups are empowered to take decisions on behalf of the board. These decisions will commit the board just as positively as if they had been taken by executive committees made up of board members. The exceptional degree of delegation, which is the basis of the present relationship between members and officers, has contributed to the role confusion experienced by board members, many of whom have found great difficulty in adjusting to an altered environment. Even the strategic planning role reserved for board members is largely influenced by the kinds of information and options supplied by officers.

Development fund allocations illustrate some of the changes described above. The extensive scale of delegation by the board to chief officers includes authority to vary staffing establishments and create new posts. Authority to create a new post is delegated to the area or district executive group on the basis that, if funds are available for an additional post, all demands for extra staff must be taken into account. The responsibility is then on the members of the group, not, as before, to present a case to the board in their individual capacities and await its decision, but to agree the right decision among themselves. In short, the boards are concerned with principles and their officers give effect to these through a wide range of detailed decisions. It is physically impossible for the small number of health boards to take, or explicitly confirm, the same number of decisions as their predecessors did collectively. The fifteen health boards replace the 150 or so bodies previously responsible for the NHS in Scotland. Moreover, the number of lay people participating in NHS administration in Scotland has been reduced from over 1500 before 1974 to 276 since then. On any count, the points at which important decisions involving lay members are made with regard to the local operation of health services have been drastically reduced. There are now only fifteen key points of decision-making which involve lay members. The combined effect of these changes is that the role of board members has contracted considerably, while the role of officers has greatly expanded. In practice, this could mean that lay members are 'restricted to a policy-approving and monitoring role, leaving detailed management and the formulation of policy' to officers (emphasis added; but see below) (32).

To seek an explanation for this shift in operating practice, it is necessary to refer to the controversy surrounding successive attempts to make a clear distinction between policy and administration. Although the debate is a somewhat sterile one, since there is ample evidence in the literature on organisations to support the conclusion that it is quite impossible to separate the two activities in view of their interrelatedness (33), this has not prevented enthusiastic reformers, often in the shape of management consultants or those with experience of private sector management practices, from indulging in numerous attempts to draw just such a distinction. The difficulties involved in trying to make a distinction are spelled out in a report on the management of local government which appeared in 1967. It says:

> 'We do not believe that it is possible to lay down what is policy and what is administrative detail; some issues stand out as important and can be regarded as 'policy'; other matters, seemingly trivial, may involve political or social reaction

> of such significance that deciding them becomes a matter of policy and members feel that they must reserve to themselves consideration and decision on them. A succession of detailed decisions may contribute, eventually, to the formulation of a policy' (34).

It is precisely because policy and administration are largely inseparable that the official circular (35) dealing with the roles of health board members and officers is vague. For example, it states that:

> 'the powers formally delegated to the executive group may vary from place to place and in practice some decisions involving few resources would be referred to the board because of their interest to the community generally whilst others involving greater use of resources but flowing naturally from decisions of principle made by the board would be taken by the executive group'.

In effect, therefore, the circular admits that it is not really possible to make a clear-cut distinction between policy and administration. But the outcome of the attempt to clarify the respective roles and functions of board members and officers has been a reduction in the contribution which board members can make to decision-making (36). Because 'policy implementation' feeds back 'into policy formation' (37) and is the basis of future policy, if board members are to be cut off from any involvement in this feedback stage (and they were involved in day-to-day management and administration before 1974), then any policies they approve will inevitably be heavily based on the advice and recommendations received from officers. What tends to happen in practice in such a situation is the exact opposite of what is intended, namely, that officers formulate the policy and board members argue about the technicalities of administering it (38).

A feature of the previous administrative structure was its 'committee-intensive' nature. This has given way to a simpler committee structure in keeping with the emphasis on the policy-making, as distinct from the executive, role of the lay members. All health boards have devised their own committee structures but, apart from minor variations, most boards have the following committees: the main one is concerned with policy and resources (some boards have separate committees for these activities); another is concerned with general purposes (i.e. personnel, staffing, manpower planning); and then there are the statutory Part IV committees for the various services, e.g. general medical, general dental and general pharmaceutical. Guidance from the SHHD on committees stated that 'the object should be to limit the number of committees as far as possible', and envisaged a policy and resource allocation committee and committees for Part IV services. The committee structure has proved a problem in many areas, mainly because of the need to involve board members in decision-making. Some boards have established a second standing committee, apart from a policy and resources one, in order to overcome this problem and to involve those board members who are not on the policy and resources committee. In certain boards, there is no practical need for a second committee, other than to make members feel involved in proceedings, and it has sometimes been difficult, because of lack of business, to draw up an agenda for a particular meeting. One of the effects of having a policy and resources committee as the major committee of a board has been to concentrate business in the hands of this committee, and to limit discussion at full board meetings. Since full board meetings are open to the press and public, this may be a contributing factor to such a development, but it creates additional difficulties for board members who are not on this committee.

In addition to these committees, health boards have also established programme planning committees, usually as sub-committees of the policy and resources or equivalent committee, to assist boards in the formulation of long term policies in regard to particular services, like primary care, and client groups, like the elderly. The membership is multidisciplinary and includes two board members, one of whom is normally chairman. These committees were only just being established when the research was undertaken, so they had no impact on the decision process investigated. However, in an examination of programme planning committees in the Greater Glasgow Health Board, Boddy (39) reports that 'overwhelmingly, the impression gained was of a group of people who were dissatisfied with the way the committees were working, and with the results obtained'.

A number of other features of the Scottish Health Service ought to be mentioned. They come under the collective heading of advice. Health care planning in Scotland is rather different from that in England, both institutionally and in approach. The Scottish Health Service Planning Council, representing all the health boards as well as university and Scottish Office interests, exists to advise the Secretary of State on the exercise of his functions, whether at his request or on its own initiative. There is no English equivalent of this body. According to its first annual report (40), the Planning Council sees itself as an important part of the central administration of the NHS with a 'key part to play in opening up new possibilities in regard to the provision of health care in Scotland'. In England, the emphasis has been on comprehensive health planning with the development of an annual planning cycle in which the centre plays a key role. In Scotland, a greater emphasis has been placed on flexibility, participation and strategic, as opposed to comprehensive, planning (41). The work of the Council is inevitably long-term in character, although reports are now emerging from the Programme Planning Groups established to focus on specific client-groups like the elderly, the mentally disordered, children and so on. The Council was also involved in approving the recommendations made in the SHHD memorandum (42), reviewing health policies and priorities for the period up to 1979/80. It will shortly be issuing planning guidelines for 1980 and beyond.

A feature of the reorganised Service is that it provides for health boards to be advised by the providers and consumers of health care. Professional consultative committees have been established by the various health care professions to represent their views at national, area and, in some boards, at district levels. Local Health Councils (LHCs) have been established to represent the public interest. In the reorganised NHS, advice is much more 'purposefully channelled' and is intended to have a greater influence on health board decision-making than was the case prior to 1974 (43).

The professional advisory machinery has the function of advising health boards and expressing the views of the professions both on policy issues and on matters of importance relating to the running of services. There is little doubt that the best organised professional advisory committees are the medical ones. The main aim of the medical advisory structure is 'to provide a channel of access to management, to express a corporate medical viewpoint, and to provide a general background of accepted medical priorities' (44).

LHCs (the Scottish equivalent of CHCs in England and Wales) stand outside the formal management structure. Their 'independence' needs to be qualified since members are, in part, appointed by health authorities, who also finance the Councils and provide them with accommodation. LHCs can offer advice and suggestions on their own initiative and they are consulted by health service managers for their views on changes in services and on future plans and proposals, including hospital closures. They have access to information to help them assess how well facilities in their districts match up to recommended standards. They are able to visit health service establishments, and are required to submit annual reports to their health authorities. LHCs perform a difficult role. To achieve the correct balance between representing the public view, as far as appointed bodies are able to do so and, at the same time, appreciating and understanding constructively the problems faced by, and the constraints operating on, management is not easy. Furthermore, the existence of LHCs has caused some confusion among board members, who regard their role in similar terms to that prescribed for LHCs.

(c) <u>The Mechanics of the Budgetary Process</u>

The total cost of services provided by health boards in Scotland is covered by an annual allocation determined by the Scottish Office, with the exception of the cost of the family practitioner services, which are not subject to any form of budgetary constraint because they are largely 'demand determined'. The mechanism for financing the health service is through the annual submission, for approval by Parliament, of the supply estimates. The estimates for the Scottish Health Service are put forward by the SHHD, independently of, but simultaneously with, the estimates for England and Wales. Separate allocations of finance are made to health boards for capital and revenue purposes, and all proposals for expenditure have to recognise this important distinction. The following discussion concentrates on revenue funds of a recurring nature, principally expenditure on staff.

Expenditure on the NHS, although globally determined, is, at the end of the day, broadly used to purchase resources in the fulfilment of priorities determined locally. Although health boards can dispose of development monies according to their own priorities, occasionally the initiative for new developments may come from the centre. For example, the decision to redeploy resources from acute services to the 'Cinderella' sectors of the NHS was taken by the centre. Therefore, the discretion of field health authorities to distribute their development funds according to their own wishes is, to some extent, circumscribed by central government policy initiatives. Furthermore, the duties and responsibilities of health boards are decided by statute which limits the purposes for which expenditure can be incurred.

These caveats apart, however, as Levitt (45) notes in regard to the DHSS, it maintains 'that only ... broad and long-term priorities can be decided centrally - it is at local level that the details of resource allocation are really determined'. The SHHD's report for 1977 (46) states that 'the deployment of revenue resources is largely determined by the decisions of individual health boards in that over 90% of the revenue monies available for running hospital and community services are distributed to them'. Brown (47) goes further and argues that 'most initiatives come from the grass roots - from the desire of people at the point of delivery for developments that would make their own work more useful, interesting, or satisfying'.

Within health boards, discretion over allocations is normally confined to the DF at their disposal and boards are free to decide upon detailed disbursements, e.g. which categories of staff require expansion: whether, for instance, maternity services should be cut back, or services for the elderly improved, and so on.

About 70% of the total expenditure on the Scottish Health Service is for current expenditure. What is significant about the entire system of resource allocation, the questioning of which has been responsible for RAWP (in England) and SHARE (in Scotland) (48), is its historical basis - the previous year's allocation determines the current year's allocation. Gentle and Forsythe (49) acknowledge that revenue has traditionally been allocated to health authorities largely in proportion to 1948 allocations. Likewise, the interim report of the SHHD's Working Party on Revenue Resource Allocation (50) notes that 'there was no conscious effort during this period (i.e. from 1948 to 1978) to effect redistribution of funds as between Regional Hospital Boards'. Nevertheless, there were continual tensions, which remain in relations between the centre and health authorities, as to whether there should be a greater earmarking of funds for various purposes, or whether boards should be allocated the maximum available money to meet local needs as they, and not central government, thought best (51). The decisive argument in favour of the latter approach was, the interim report (52) suggests, 'that earmarked funds often remained unspent because there was no way of transferring them to other purposes quickly enough to enable the total ... allocation of the board to be used by the end of the financial year'.

Although there is still concern at the persistence of uneven patterns of expenditure, and despite national policy guidelines which favour a shift of resources from acute services to services for the chronic sick and the mentally ill, earmarking is not seen as a solution to these imbalances. Instead, the intention (as outlined in RAWP and SHARE) is to shift the pattern by moving funds in the direction of the authorities with the greater needs (the definition of 'need' being one of the more thorny of the problems tackled by the two working parties). The implications of this shift, planned to take effect over a ten year period beginning in 1978-9, are that historical patterns of resource allocation will be broken.

> 'The major change of emphasis in SHARE as compared with the previous method of distributing resources to the areas is that the sole basis for allocation is what the different areas need. Previously - and illogically - the basis of allocation was heavily influenced by what the area had by way of health care facilities. Historical inertia modified only by the loudest voice is no way to determine such an important matter as the fair distribution of health care expenditures'(53).

Of course, RAWP and SHARE are concerned with whether the national development cake is being divided most equitably between health authorities; they are not concerned with the purposes upon which boards spend their allocations.

A constraint on the freedom of health boards to allocate resources and plan expenditure was that, until quite recently, revenue allocations were fixed in that they had to be used in the particular financial year for which they were provided. This method of financing gave rise to criticism that it produced year-end spending sprees, or 'Christmas handouts'. However, a limited degree of flexibility in the use of fixed financial allocations has been introduced which has made it possible to carry forward small unspent balances from one financial year to the next (up to 1%). This has not eliminated the 'Christmas handout' syndrome although it has reduced both its occurrence and the size of the sums of money involved.

Outside the field of major capital expenditures (where central sanction is required for new schemes), central influence in the NHS is largely geared to dealing with classes of local issues rather than with specific local issues. In short, most central control is 'contextuating' rather than 'prescriptive' - central government is primarily concerned with setting contexts for local operations through formulating generic policy positions (54).

The very nature of the structure of the NHS, and the method by which it is financed from the centre, makes the likelihood of a tension-free relationship between centre and periphery remote. The NHS comprises a plurality of field authorities, spending large sums of money and operating with considerable independence for most of the time. But because all these authorities are also answerable to a political head accountable to Parliament, the central department feels compelled to involve itself in matters involving resources, such as changes of use for hospitals, or hospital closures. Because these are highly contentious issues it is important that the SHHD should be able to explain what is happening in the event of parliamentary questions being asked. It is also essential that the Department remain accountable to Parliament through the Secretary of State for the way in which funds voted for the NHS are spent.

The budgetary process and the relationship between centre, (SHHD), and periphery, (health boards), are virtually inseparable. The process by which resources are allocated to boards, and the extent to which the centre is involved in the use of these resources, reveals the amount of discretion boards possess to pursue their own priorities as determined at the local level. Boards have, in theory at any rate but also in practice to a considerable degree, a large amount of autonomy to allocate monies, although in times of economic uncertainty, when there is concern about escalating public expenditure, the centre can be expected, understandably in the circumstances, to intervene more directly in the affairs of health authorities. However, financial considerations are not the only relevant factors affecting central - local relations. Hence the value of the concept of 'power-dependence' (55) which directs attention to the 'reciprocal nature of power relationships'. As Rhodes (56) observes in the context of local government, 'no matter how great the power of a central department over a local authority, it is still dependent to some degree on that local authority'.

The obstacles standing in the way of the development of a mutually acceptable relationship between centre and periphery stem largely from the fact that the structure of the NHS rests on an attempt to reconcile the irreconcilable. The twin features of the structure, centralism and localism, are dichotomous. The dilemma at the root of the dichotomy is that if, on the one hand, health authorities are to be left to choose how they distribute their funds, then national priorities run the risk of becoming little more than rhetorical exercises. But if, on the other hand, central government is to determine priorities then local initiatives and autonomy are, at the very least, severely curtailed. As an observer (57) of the DHSS planning system for the NHS in England has written: 'the unknown in the question remains: to what extent will local health authorities be free to interpret in their own way the policy guidelines offered by the Department?'

In Scotland, too, the interplay between centre and periphery is a recurring theme in any analysis of resource-allocation, and later chapters return to it when some of the <u>external</u> constraints impinging on those charged with allocating DF are examined. However, it is also worth noting that while health boards may possess a degree of autonomy to allocate resources (particularly DF) and decide priorities, their ability in practice to enjoy this freedom is circumscribed by numerous <u>internal</u> constraints which can have a more potent impact on the decision process within health boards than attempts by the centre to impose its will.

CHAPTER 3

Theoretical Approaches and Research Setting

The making of decisions is a fundamental part of every human activity and, at its simplest, may be perceived as the selection of one specific course of action from among two or more alternatives, that is, as a process involving some kind of choice. The adequacy of this view has been challenged by the introduction of the notion of a 'non-decision' (1). It is worth exploring this concept a little further since, as will be shown in Chapters 4 and 5, the constraints operating on decision-makers were such that a very narrow range of options was in fact open to them; indeed, some possibilities did not even find their way on to the agenda. Therefore, non-decision-making might be a more appropriate term to describe what was happening than decision-making, if the latter is taken to mean the unfettered freedom to select a particular course of action (i.e. without being subject to numerous constraints which serve to restrict the choices available). Dubin (2) has summarised the argument well:

> 'Decisions are made to guide the course of human action. Two general outcomes of decisions are possible: 1) to select a new course of action different from that being pursued; and 2) to choose the present course of action as the best among available alternatives, thus continuing ongoing activities unchanged'.

Dearlove (3), in his study of policy-making in one local authority, concludes that the decisional activity observed was restricted 'to the making of routine decisions involving the maintenance of established commitments ...'. As this statement suggests, non-decision-making, which is basically what Dearlove means in his use of the term 'policy maintenance', can be included in definitions of decision-making. In fact, following the work of Bachrach and Baratz (4), Parry and Morriss (5) argue that:

> 'non-decisions are decisions. They are not, however, necessarily the sorts of 'key decisions' studied by the 'decisional approach' associated with the work of Dahl and his associates. Many are lesser decisions which are component parts of a routine and the power which a routine reflects may be of a different kind to that discovered by the analysis of decisions'.

In essence, Parry and Morriss advocate a decisional approach to non-decisions, whereby the definition of a non-decision begins by stating that it is a decision. This extension of the term decision-making to include the notion of non-decision-making is useful if an attempt is being made, as it is here, to penetrate a particular decision process with a view to understanding more fully precisely what is involved, i.e. to see which of Dubin's decision outcomes best fits the process observed and to discover why.

The political nature of decision-making was noted in Chapter 1, although it is necessary to be clear about what is understood by the term 'political'. Klein's (6) view that 'politics are ... about the reconciliation of conflicting interests' (emphasis added) is misleading, if this is all that is embraced by the term. Politics are also about the operation of routines, standard operating procedures (SOPs) (7) and conflict avoidance. Yet decision-making of this routine variety is a neglected part of politics. Parry and Morriss believe that while politics are a matter of decisions and choices, they are also 'a matter of customs and regulations ...' (8). In their discussion of routines and SOPs, Parry and Morriss draw on the work of Sharkansky (9) and Lukes (10). In his analysis of power, Lukes is anxious to show that non-decision-making need not involve 'actual, observable conflict, overt or covert' (11). According to Lukes (12) 'A may exercise power over B by getting him to do what he does not want to do, but he also exercises power over him by influencing, shaping or determining his very wants'. This agenda-setting role, which operates to prevent conflict from arising in the first place, has received insufficient attention in studies of decision-making. What is valuable about Lukes' analysis for present purposes is his attempt to perceive non-decision-making as an activity which can occur through organisational routines and through social forces operating outwith the particular system being observed. As the case study will reveal, decisions on the allocation of DF involved few clear instances of actual conflict and emerged from a mix of precedent and institutional practices. Many of the constraints operating on the two health boards arose not from within the health service but from elsewhere, including local authorities. In a number of cases, particular allocation decisions were the outcome, albeit indirectly, of decisions taken by local authorities.

The adherence to routines was not simply the result of issues being kept off the agenda, or being decided elsewhere. It was also the outcome of puzzlement on the part of decision-makers as to what they should be doing and how they should be doing it. Heclo (13), for instance, maintains that references to competing claims should not be taken to imply that all, or even the predominant feature of, social politics is conflict and the play of power. Because the issues faced in social politics are so complex, the major difficulty may be not the exercise of political will, but the determination of what that will is, or ought to be. In other words, the situation confronting decision-makers may be less one of competing for power and more one of coping with uncertainty, or the 'possibly unwinnable dilemmas of social policy' (14).

Heclo's view of power and decision-making would appear to be of some relevance to the process observed in the two health boards. While the power factor may have had a bearing on the process, in particular the relationship between administrators and health care professionals (15), perhaps more in evidence were the constraints and uncertainties surrounding decision-makers in a setting where there are no clear measures of output or performance. Output measures based on numbers of inpatient admissions or days of care are, as one commentator (16) has argued, 'conceptually inadequate when what we ought to be discussing is the tangible contribution made to people's health'. Qualitative measures of this kind, however, are notoriously difficult to devise. In the words of one health board Secretary (17) it is 'extremely difficult, if not impossible, to say that additional input X led directly to improvement in health status Y'. Allied to this is the difficulty of actually knowing when an objective has been met; for example, what level of service provision constitutes an adequate level of care for the elderly? Or when is it possible to say that enough has been provided in the way of services for the mentally disordered? Heclo expresses the dilemma succinctly: 'social politics arises because men disagree among themselves, but also because they do not know what to do or how to do it' (18). To this extent, policy <u>results</u> - it does not get <u>made</u> (19). Rivlin (20) reaches a similar conclusion in her claim that social problems remain unsolved:

> 'because we do not know how to do it ... The difficulties do not primarily involve conflicts among different groups of people, although these exist. Rather, current social problems are difficult because they involve conflicts among objectives that almost everyone holds'.

A study of decision-making, including the notion of non-decision-making, from such a perspective may be conveyed by the term <u>administrative politics</u> (21). According to Self (22), 'administrative politics revolve around the discretionary decisions of administrative agencies or departments'. There has been an expansion of these with the growth of public agencies and, it might be added, the managerial bias of the reorganisation of the NHS, which has transferred much specific policy-making to the administrative arena (23).

Having established that the term decision-making can be used to include non-decision-making (on the basis that to do nothing is still the outcome of choice), and that it refers to the routines and SOPs, which collectively form a system of administrative politics, adopted by administrative agencies, partly in response to power relations but also in response to uncertainty, it remains to examine theories of decision-making for their ability to make sense of a particular decision process by alerting an investigator to the features which seem most important and by providing plausible accounts of events.

THEORIES OF DECISION-MAKING

In the literature on decision-making, the study of the act of choice has focused on: (1) the origins of the decision (where the issue that had to be resolved originated from); (2) the procedures by which the decision was made; (3) the influence of the background of the decision-makers themselves on the choices they make; (4) the influence of the institutional or organisational environment on the decisions; and (5) the content of the decision itself. Different theories of decision-making have highlighted some of these variables at the expense of others.

The concept of administrative politics, introduced earlier, directs a researcher to an exploration of the internal mechanisms of organisations which does not simply focus upon the action, or inaction, of individual decision-makers but also upon their interaction with the organisational environment of which they form a part. Such a perspective leads naturally to an examination of incremental theories of decision-making to ascertain their relevance for providing insights into, and helping to account for, the way in which a particular decision process proceeds as it does. However, a discussion of incrementalism cannot precede consideration of rational theories. Although the emergence of incrementalist theories was, in part, a reaction to the rather monolithic, mechanistic and one-dimensional approach of the rationalists who were primarily concerned with how organisations should function rather than with how they in fact operated, rational theories are also relevant in furthering an understanding of organisational phenomena. Reference to them is unavoidable if for no other reason than their persistence among some organisational reformers (e.g. management consultants). Of course, there exist multiple perceptions of rationality in the NHS where each individual, or group, may believe that he, or they, are acting rationally in the sense of maximising his, or their, interests. For example, doctors share a concept of rationality that appertains to standards of care for individual patients, whereas administrators view rationality as linked to equity of service provision and the most economic use of resources (24). Moreover, for different levels of organisation (e.g. areas and districts) it may be rational for those administering them to argue for the best possible levels of service provision, even if by doing so the attempt to equalise service provision throughout an area may be made that much harder to achieve. This notion of rationality was a feature of the two health boards observed, and it influenced attempts by the areas to achieve savings (25). However, for present purposes, rationality as an ideal type of decision-making refers to the application of a set of specific procedures which are most likely to achieve optimal decisions in terms of a particular set of aims or objectives.

The pursuit of rationality, in this specifically normative sense, was instrumental in the design of the NHS management arrangements. Self (26), noting 'the managerial belief in paradigms of rational decision-making', has argued that organisations may need to be drastically changed to facilitate the rational approach. As Self (27) makes clear, 'it does not follow that ... managerial ... aims are intrinsically 'wrong' but that the results of such reforms may not accord with expectations'. It is at the interface of rational theories, (which largely govern the present structural shape of the NHS), and incremental theories, (which can account for departures from rationality and for distortions of the management structure), that many of the tensions described in later chapters arise (28). It is, therefore, fruitful to explore from different perspectives, that is, the rational, the incremental and the various dimensions within each, the numerous tensions and conflicts which may be present in a decision process.

(a) <u>Rationality</u>

Although the classical theorists of rationality (e.g. Taylor's 'scientific management') (29) are somewhat discredited in much current organisation theory literature, 'many management experts who advise governments today use a somewhat similar approach and assumptions' (30).

The rational model is based on three stages which are considered to be necessary in the realisation of a rationally calculated decision: (1) the decision-maker considers all of the alternatives (courses of action) open to him; (2) he identifies and evaluates all of the consequences which would flow from the adoption of each alternative; and (3) he selects that alternative the probable consequences of which would be preferable in terms of his most valued ends. Above all, a rational decision entails clarity, and agreement, about goals and objectives, and a search for the best possible means of attaining them. Every possible strategy should be reviewed, so that the best can be selected, and decision-makers should guard against undesirable side-effects by studying all the possible consequences of each. The development, and application, of management techniques like cost-benefit analysis, programme-planning-budgeting, management by objectives, operational research, corporate planning and, more recently, zero-based budgeting illustrates the successive attempts by reformers to find ways to bring decision-making more in line with the rational model (31). Although these techniques are supposed to enable a rational choice to be made among a range of alternatives, in fact, as Edwards III and Sharkansky confirm, few of the techniques make an impact on actual decisions for the simple reason that 'the demands of rational analysis are simply too great despite the sincerest efforts to achieve it'(32).

Ideas associated with rationality, and some of the techniques stemming from it, have been incorporated into the management arrangements of the reorganised NHS. For instance, the changed relationship between health board members and officers considered in the last chapter is a consequence of a commitment to a managerial (i.e. rational) model of reform. The uplifted role of the Treasurer is also significant since he is entrusted with the task of introducing, and applying, many of the techniques associated with rationality, such as management accounting, position statements and output budgets. There is also an attempt in the NHS to shift the emphasis from a concern with inputs to a concern with outputs as decision-makers strive to utilise resources more efficiently and effectively. In the case of the medical profession, where interference by administrators is resisted, Community Medicine Specialists (CMSs) are expected to inject some rationality into decisions taken by doctors at the sharp end of the Service. The training of CMSs places considerable (some would argue too much) emphasis upon the measurement of need and cost, and upon the assessment of priorities through epidemiological methodology (33). Another instance of the application of rationality in the reorganised NHS concerns the creation of consensus management teams whose task it is to examine the needs of the Service comprehensively in a corporate fashion, and then act unanimously.

The emphasis on management in the reorganised NHS may be contrasted with the administration of the Service before its reform. A distinction between the two activities, management and administration, is useful in order to illuminate the subtle differences in practice since 1974, although not too much ought to be made of the distinction since both terms are, in practice, used interchangeably (34). Administration is a more limited form of activity than management and is less concerned with advocating change than with implementing policy and achieving stability through the maintenance of existing practices and procedures. Management, however, is more about promoting change, a conception which has some validity if the stress on this activity in the NHS since reorganisation is viewed as being motivated primarily by a desire to plan the Service so as to enable quite dramatic shifts to occur in health care policy, in particular a shift from hospital-based to community-based care (35). In short, administration refers to the operation of routines within a prevailing infrastructure of health service policies and institutional arrangements, while management refers to attempts to alter the infrastructure rather than merely the superstructure.

A rational model, as Allison (36), among others, has suggested, presupposes the existence of a consensus within an organisation among those involved in taking decisions. The commitment to consensus management within the NHS illustrates the belief in rationality which underlay much of the thinking at the time of reorganisation. Basically, the greater the degree of rationality in a decision process, the greater the emphasis on consensus, on harmony, on a corporate approach to decision-making and on 'technical' criteria for the evaluation of proposals; conversely, the less the degree of rationality, the greater the emphasis on political 'wheeling and dealing' and incrementalism (37). Allison's rational actor model (RAM) sees choices in any field of decision-making as being clearly defined and based on rational assessments of public desires - it is simply a matter of fulfilling well-defined goals in an optimal manner. Decisions taken within the framework of the RAM reflect a single, coherent and consistent set of calculations about particular problems. The possibility of organisational and political complications fouling the smooth-running machine simply do not enter into the model's orbit, largely because rational models are normative and prescriptive rather than descriptive.

Nevertheless, although of limited value in illuminating how decisions are taken, and although inclined to obscure rather than to reveal, an appreciation of rationality can further our understanding of the operations of organisations. As already noted, the present structure of the NHS is largely derived from rational theories. These assume a unitary view of organisational relationships (hence the emphasis on consensus) within the Service, and that all those making decisions identify with, and share in, a common, superordinate goal, that is, the welfare of patients. Tensions, or clashes of interest, are perceived as irrational and are defined as 'technical' problems, for example, a failure in communication, poor information, and so on. This line of reasoning lay behind much of the diagnosis of the problems which existed within the pre-1974 model of the NHS, in particular the lack of co-ordination between the three arms of the Service (38).

Dimmock and Barnard (39) have commented on the degree to which assumptions of a unitary perspective permeated the reorganisation of the NHS, particularly in the adoption of the concept of consensus management by multidisciplinary teams. Yet, as the authors are well aware, the true picture to emerge from the upheaval of reorganisation is more complicated. Dimmock and Barnard (40) observe that:

> 'the Service appeared to espouse the simple unitary view that the objective of Reorganisation, though about management, was in the interests of the patient ... (But) the outcomes (of the new arrangements) were significantly influenced by the need to reconcile conflicting interests rather than by some sense of an optimum structure determined by the patients' needs'.

The unitary perspective 'has denied the existence of sectional interests and, in consequence, has largely failed to provide an accurate description of inter-group relationships within the Service or relationships with the external environment'(41). The authors advocate an alternative perspective with which to view the NHS, one which acknowledges the pluralism of such organisations where groups coexist, each having its own objectives. To pursue this further, it is necessary to introduce incrementalist theories of decision-making.

(b) Incrementalism

Incrementalist theories of decision-making are most closely associated with the writings of Lindblom (42). The 'strategy of muddling through' is directed towards the solution of immediate, pressing problems rather than with the realisation of some distant goal. Muddling through attacks these immediate problems incrementally, that is, through a consideration of alternative policies which differ only marginally from current policies. This immediately restricts the number of alternatives considered, making the problem of choice more manageable. Choice may be aided, too, because prediction of the consequences of these marginal changes may be more feasible and it may also be easier for decision-makers to evaluate a range of policies where these involve only marginal change from the existing base-line. Therefore, progress is made through a continual process of 'partisan mutual adjustment'.

A further characteristic of the strategy is that analysis and decision-making are seen as fragmented activities, undertaken by different agencies in a disjointed manner, hence the term 'disjointed incrementalism'. Insofar as there were observable divisions between area and district tiers in the two health boards, which hindered efforts at synoptic problem-solving at area level, then elements of this primary meaning of 'disjointed' were indeed evident (43). But the notion of 'disjointedness' also has a secondary meaning which is of greater relevance for the case study. Braybrooke and Lindblom (44) state that decision-making may be disjointed in a secondary sense because of its focus on 'remedial policies that "happen" to be at hand rather than addressing (itself) to a more comprehensive set of goals and alternative policies'.

There are strong similarities between incrementalism and Simon's (45) notions of 'bounded rationality' and 'satisficing' which, since there are cognitive limits on rationality, account more precisely for the way in which decisions are reached in practice. In his analysis of foreign policy decision-making, Allison (46) has developed models derived from an incrementalist perspective. In his book, he utilises two models, the Organisational Process Model and the Governmental Politics Model, but elsewhere (47) combines the two models to form the Bureaucratic Politics Model (BPM). This model views decisions not as the outcome of consensus and harmony but as the outcome of a series of bargaining games. There is no unitary mode of action but rather a pluralistic mode, where there is no single strategy for solving a particular problem but many strategies. Organisations are made up of disparate, decentralised units in which the actors perform with different perspectives and priorities, and decisions are made by much pulling and hauling among them, and not by a single rational choice as in the RAM. The BPM is also concerned with how certain patterns of activity take place in an organisation, focusing on the pattern of statements, directives and actions of the relevant departments and parts of an organisation including the adoption of bargaining strategies, tactics, conventions (rules of the game), routines, standard operation procedures (SOPs), and so on.

Dimmock and Barnard's (48) pluralist view of organisations shares a similar focus on the perspectives of individual actors in any decision process.

> 'The pluralist view sees organisations as containing a number of related but separate interests and objectives which must be maintained in some kind of equilibrium. Instead of the concept of a corporate unity reflected in one source of authority and loyalty, there exist rival sources of leadership and attachment'.

The authors acknowledge the fact that 'to date the health field has neither admitted nor subscribed to analyses of organisational behaviour which point to the existence of conflicts of interest and the pursuit of sectional interests'(49).

Incrementalism perceives decision-making as a political activity, where proposals and decisions are to the advantage of some but inevitably, too, to the disadvantage of others. It also acknowledges the importance of institutional structures within which decision-making is undertaken. These are characterised by divisions of tasks faced by an organisation into separate predefined parts; duties are allocated to different positions. The rational, or unitary, model assumes that these separate divisions interlock efficiently, as in Weber's view of bureaucracy with its division of labour and commitment to hierarchy, in order that a comprehensive and coherent range of instruments can be developed to realise given aims. But an incrementalist, or pluralist, model views these organisational divisions somewhat differently. The notion of 'divisions' refers to political and/or organisational differences, where actors have conflicting loyalties rather than share an overriding loyalty to the organisation as a whole. It has been suggested (50) that the major failures of comprehensive planning stem from its definition of comprehensiveness in a world that lacks any comprehensive political power or institutions.

The theory of incremental decision-making is often put forward as an explanation of budgetary processes (51). Indeed, Ball (52) and Allison (53) argue that budgets and procurement decisions are likely to be more amenable than other types to explanation in terms of bureaucratic politics. In his classic study of budgetary processes, Wildavsky (54) set out to construct a theory of the formation of the Federal budget based on a detailed description of the decision process surrounding it. While emphasising the complexity of the budget-maker's problem, Wildavsky describes a series of 'aids to calculation' to help decision-makers simplify a problem and reach a decision (55). Wildavsky's theory is consistent with Lindblom's: emphasis is placed upon the limited capacity of individuals to comprehend the full complexities of their environment. Because of the impossibility of exploring all available alternatives, reality has to be simplified to enable a decision-maker to realise a choice. As March and Simon (56) argue, the rationality of classical 'economic man', who makes 'optimal' choices in a clearly defined environment, gives way to the rationality of 'administrative man', who satisfices in place of discovering and selecting optimal alternatives.

Greenwood <u>et al</u> (57) are critical of explanations of budgetary processes that emphasise 'bounded rationality' and 'satisficing'. They accept that these notions of incrementalism contain a great deal of plausibility, and agree that probably all budgetary processes are incremental in that most of budget goes unexamined in any single year. The two health boards chosen for the research proved to be no exception. The authors also accept that one of the reasons for the lack of a comprehensive review is probably the limited information handling capabilities, and finite intellectual abilities, of decision-makers. But the weakness, in their view, of this

> 'limited rationality thesis ... is its inability to explain why some budgetary processes are <u>more or less incremental than other budgetary processes</u>. The implication is that incrementalism could be avoided, or reduced, by increasing the intellectual capacity of budgetary actors, or by reducing the complexity of the information at his disposal (e.g. by using a computer)(58) (emphasis added)'.

Cornford (59) shares some of these misgivings but goes further, claiming that 'there is much in government which is not incremental and much that may be incremental in appearance though not in consequences'. Furthermore, he maintains that 'disjointed incrementalism ... <u>exaggerates the degree of stability and regularity</u> in government'(60) (emphasis added), a view also held by Ruggie (61) who believes that incrementalism over-simplifies social complexity and decision-making processes through its sequential ordering of events and procedures and their individual marginal adjustment. In short, incrementalism may carry with it the danger of imputing to decision-making a degree of orderliness and continuity which is, in fact, not present.

Greenwood <u>et al</u> propose an adapted incrementalist model which incorporates some of the inchoateness of political processes which can operate at random, often according to the dictates of fashion (62). The authors maintain that because

> 'budgets are the outcome of clashes between entrenched interests ... a more adequate theory of budgeting ... will have to be based upon the political features of organisational life, rather than upon the cognitive deficiencies of decision actors'(63).

The authors are critical of Wildavsky's approach because although he is aware of 'the politics of organisational life', his explanation of the budgetary process fails to capture this dimension. Only by examining organisational politics, (synonymous with the notion of administrative politics introduced earlier), is it possible to account for why some budgetary processes are more incremental than others. To meet their objective, Greenwood et al present a set of concepts designed to capture organisational politics. The concepts are concerned with (i) the impact of the environment on decision processes, (ii) organisational characteristics and arrangements, and (iii) the interests, values and power of those groups comprising an organisation. They are germane to the case study since it would appear from the study that the scope for change is a product of the very political processes within organisations that Greenwood et al are anxious to open up. For instance, reference has been made to the intention within parts of the NHS to shift priority from acute services to non-acute ones. Of this policy initiative, one health board Secretary has written (64)

> 'the current emphasis on the non-acute aspects of health care may be the correct one but it is difficult to avoid the conclusion that it owes more to political judgement - if not hunch - than to any objective assessment of needs and resources'.

Greenwood et al, as Judge (65) points out, have not discarded the concept of incrementalism but have added substantially to it in an attempt to overcome some of the criticisms levelled at it. Nevertheless, Judge is not wholly persuaded by the authors' analysis and attempt at revisionism, and suggests that perhaps they 'exaggerate the occurrence of overt conflict between sub-units for resources', paying insufficient attention to the fact that 'organisational procedures minimise opportunities for open conflict'(66) (emphasis added). Routines and SOPs, as mentioned earlier, are a key element in Allison's BPM and they also feature in Danziger's (67) study of local authority budgeting in England. Clashes between entrenched interests need not always actually occur - mere anticipation of them may be sufficient for decision-makers to attempt to avoid, or minimise, them. This line of reasoning recalls the discussion of Lukes' work and, specifically, his concept of latent conflict 'which consists in a contradiction between the interests of those exercising power and the real interests of those they exclude'(68). Moreover, recalling also the discussion earlier of the presence of puzzlement in social policy-making, it is important not to overlook this factor. Its influence may be unrelated either to overt, or to latent, conflict but may result in incremental decision-making all the same. Cornford (69) expresses appositely the very real paradox that exists between the operation of routines in a decision process, and the degree of uncertainty and puzzlement that is also present. Although his remarks are directed at governmental decision-making, they are equally applicable to the NHS.

> 'We may have to accept that any modern government is an incoherent system. A system because, while there is muddle, the pattern of its activities is not random; most of the conditions and constraints within which it operates have some stability over time; and there is also a degree of stability in the behaviour of its component parts. Incoherent both because there is muddle and because the pattern of events is in fact and in principle unpredictable by participants. The complexity of events is too great for them to grasp what is going on and they do not know how they themselves are going to act. If ... we mean anything by decision-making other than the illusion of choice, it must involve some element of chance' (emphases added).

THE APPLICATION OF THEORY

Klein (70) has noted that different modes of explanation have variable explanatory power, depending on the issues involved and suggests that 'to talk about theories in the plural presupposes that different modes of explanation are not necessarily mutually exclusive, and that their explanatory power may vary with the situation to which they are applied'. He seems to be saying that different issues require different modes of explanation rather than that different modes of explanation may be used to explore a particular issue. From the foregoing discussion of rationality and incrementalism as aids in understanding decision processes, it can be concluded that it is necessary to adopt both perspectives if a more complete picture of these processes is to emerge. Rein (71) in his work on public policy is concerned with searching for a way of assimilating the insights provided by different paradigms, and for him the answer lies in a multi-paradigmatic perspective with which to understand events and to interpret policy. 'Many paradigms contain stories which describe intrinsically good ways of looking at reality ... These are persuasive whether or not we accept the whole paradigm of thought from which they come (72). Rein likens the process to story-telling, which 'extracts the insights of particular paradigms from the paradigm itself and thus makes possible a multi-paradigmatic approach to policy analysis'(73).

As already mentioned, rational models of decision-making are limited since, as Dror (74) claims, they ignore extra-rational processes (that is, extra-rational in terms of an ideal-type model of rationality). The existence of these requires no elaboration. If rationality prevailed, then the NHS would not suffer from the gross resource imbalances between, and within, regions and between specialties which have persisted since the NHS began despite successive attempts to remove them culminating in a resource-allocation formula, RAWP (75), designed to halt the historical basis of health service spending. Furthermore, the overview of the NHS presented in the last chapter described a fragmented decision-making environment with many competing interests, as opposed to a unified, comprehensive one. Also Klein's analysis (76) of macro-decision-making in the NHS is indicative of a low degree of rationality.

Yet, as has already been noted, adherence to a rational paradigm, through a strong emphasis on management skills and techniques, played a central role in the design of the structure which emerged in 1974. Therefore, the decision-making environment in the two health boards observed, certainly from a structural standpoint, largely reflected the concerns of a rational model: for example, the emphasis on role clarity and precision; the commitment to 'delegation downwards' matched with 'accountability upwards'(77); and the creation of consensus management teams. For these reasons alone, the notion of rationality cannot be dismissed as being of no value in an attempt to comprehend particular decision processes. Furthermore, as Cornford (78) points out, a rational model of decision-making

> 'may not yield a satisfactory account of the policy process, but it is nevertheless part of it, since it underlies the public language in which politicians must argue and provides the legitimation of their bargains from whatever motives and interests these result'.

Much the same may be said of managers and professionals in the NHS engaged in resource-allocation. Cornford (79) goes on to suggest that

> 'even if every ... official cared only for the advancement of his personal ... or bureaucratic interest, even if all policy represents a compromise among those interests, (he) would still be obliged to argue in the language of (a rational model) of the national interest (since some approximation of the model underlies much of (his) own understanding and judgement of politics)'.

The rational model, then, may be said to be relevant in analyses of decision-making for four reasons: (1) many administrators believe they act rationally and that decisions they make are rational; (2) the model is useful as an ideal to which many decision-makers aspire, consequently it permeates their thinking to some degree and possibly governs some of their actions; (3) rationality is a legitimising characteristic - it 'provides the legitimation of ... bargains from whatever motives and interests these result'(80); and (4) concepts derived from the model can account for the particular structures inhabited by decision-makers.

Of course, a more rational budgetary review process, by which is meant the formulation of clear policy statements of objectives which are related to expenditure proposals, will not necessarily produce less incremental decisions (81). To some extent agencies have adopted management techniques to create an impression of efficiency and rationality, but whether the techniques have been fully implemented, or operating as intended, remains doubtful. Danziger (82) provides evidence to support his contention that the use of management techniques 'is rather more image than substance', with techniques like PPB having been instituted 'without ever being actually implemented in a meaningful fashion'. A more subtle explanation of the failure of management techniques to introduce rationality into decision-making is, according to Danziger, the fact that 'perhaps ... management techniques actually do tend to produce more incremental budgetary decisions ... It is possible that 'rationalising' the budgetary process alters the decision structure in a manner that makes reallocation less likely'(83). By increasing the visibility of a decision process and by allowing many more individuals and groups access to it, it is possible that this 'array of factors might increase the possibility of conflict among budgetary actors'(84). Strategies are then deployed to avoid, or minimise, conflict. Danziger found in his study of four English county boroughs (85), 'that the more "rationalised" budgetary process generated more rather than less incremental decisions'. In their study of public spending in Britain, Heclo and Wildavsky (86) reached a similar conclusion.

What Danziger's argument clearly shows is that mere instrumental devices alone cannot alter the behaviour of the decision-making environment as much as the environment can distort the operation of these devices (87). Unless a consensus over priorities, objectives, and so on can be reached then it is unlikely that management techniques can achieve much by way of innovative shifts in policy. Unless, as Allison puts it, there is a 'single, coherent, consistent'(88) view about particular problems and how they might be tackled, then the techniques are of little value in themselves. This conclusion suggests the importance of a second dimension of rationality. So far, normative, or objective, rationality has been considered and its relevance for understanding decision-making assessed. But there is also descriptive, or subjective, rationality relative to a particular frame of reference or set of perceptions of reality. Here, as was pointed out early on in the chapter, rationality takes on a multi-faceted perspective where each individual, or group, in an organisation may believe that he, or they, are acting rationally in the sense of maximising his, or their, own interests. This phenomenological approach to the notion of rationality is important since, as March and Simon (89) stress, classical organisation theory 'failed to make explicit this subjective and relative character of rationality ...' and consequently overlooked 'the organisational and social environment in which the decision maker finds himself (and which) determines what consequences he will anticipate, what ones he will not; what alternatives he will consider, what ones he will ignore'.

In addition to the adoption of a conceptual lens based on multiple notions of rationality through which to view health authorities in the NHS, it is necessary to adopt a conceptual lens based on notions of incrementalism. Incrementalism has no place in situations where the past is of no importance, where decision-makers all act as one united group with no bargaining or compromises to be forged, or where politics has no place in decision-making (in other words, where a rational model is applicable and can satisfactorily account for events). But the NHS, as subsequent chapters set out to show, is not such an environment. Incrementalism can, of course, be interpreted in different ways. Earlier it was shown how one interpretation stresses cognitive deficiencies of decision-makers and the technical problems arising from poor, or non-existent, information, while another interpretation stresses the political and organisational dimensions inherent in decision processes where conflict and clashes of interests are emphasised (although these can operate on a covert, as well as overt, level). While accepting that elements of both these perspectives are valuable, it is felt that other dimensions that have been omitted by these interpretations of incrementalism should be incorporated in any examination of decision-making. For instance, as has been argued, political and organisational dynamics are not just about conflict; they are also about routines and SOPs. Moreover, decision-making can be about puzzlement rather than about power and even if about power, this need not always be a straightforward overt A has power over B type configuration, but may operate in more subtle ways. The overriding concern, then, is to assimilate these competing approaches in such a way that an understanding of a particular process can emerge which captures as much as possible of what happened.

The adoption of a dual theoretical perspective (incorporating notions of rationality and of incrementalism) directs attention to the shape of the organisational structure, to the organisational procedures and routines in operation and to the interplay between the various participants in the process. Each perspective raises particular types of questions and asking the right questions is an essential prerequisite to obtaining meaningful answers.

The usefulness of theories and models in structuring a complex environment can lead to exaggerations of their potential. In his analysis of Allison's models, Cornford (90) claims that in each case the simplification necessary to understand complex phenomena distorts our conception of the reassembled whole. In one case (the RAM), collective values, intentions and motives are exaggerated, in the other (the BPM), their reality is denied, and

> 'both overestimate the consistency, the regularities, of the world they describe. If one imagines the governmental process as lying somewhere between a battle and a game of chess, these models begin and end too near to the orderly ..., rule bound, and reflective world of chess'(91).

The terms 'incremental' and 'muddling through' are frequently employed to describe decision-making, whether in government or in large-scale organisations. But incrementalism does not satisfactorily capture the irregularities present in, or the unpredictability of, decision making. As noted earlier, a major flaw is the linearity implicit in this class of theories which assumes a sequential progression of decisions aimed at solving particular problems marginally but with a sense of direction. In the real world there is often more confusion and uncertainty than is allowed for. In contrast to the complexity of decision-making, models and theories are simple and one-dimensional. Dror (92) argues that decision-making is not necessarily deterministic, which is the implicit assumption certainly of rationality and perhaps of incrementalism too; it is partly probabilistic and partly arbitrary.

In the attempt to understand the decision process selected for the case study, an emphasis has been placed on the participants' explanations of why things happened as they did or did not happen. This is not to assert that an adequate account of the process will necessarily emerge from the disparate accounts of different participants in that process, but rather to reaffirm the view that studies which aim to discover why participants acted in particular ways may be best conducted by focusing on the actions, or inactions, of these actors and their explanations. Such a phenomenological perspective has much to commend it. Explanations derived from this perspective, according to Carrier and Kendall (93),

> 'should be sought in terms of members' 'knowledge of society and its social problems'. Recognition is then given to the 'different frames of reference, different perspectives of reality ... different versions of the issues at stake' which are involved in the policy-making process'.

RETROSPECT

The first part of the chapter has been concerned with examining the theoretical considerations which underlie the case study. While acknowledging that incrementalist theory, and its derivatives like the bureaucratic politics perspective, perhaps best enabled a researcher to describe what was being observed, it was stressed that since assumptions of rationality had been a prominent feature of the management arrangements to emerge from reorganisation then notions of rationality could not be jettisoned.

For these, and other, reasons it was felt that a more flexible use of competing models, or paradigms, would be appropriate, especially if a perspective is adopted which attaches importance to 'comprehending the actors' view of reality ...'(94). Moreover, as Klein (95) points out, all 'tools of explanation ... explain <u>something</u>; none explains everything'. Through the adoption of this mixed, eclectic approach (i.e. combining insights derived from rational and incrementalist perspectives as well as from notions of puzzlement and uncertainty) it is hoped that this will make for a richer, deeper profile of a particular decision process. Rein's concept of story-telling, which draws on insights provided by numerous paradigms and attempts to relate these to events being observed in order better to understand them, makes it clear that some kind of theoretical framework is essential as a guide for moving about the field in a reasonably coherent manner. This rather loosely structured, 'open' analytical approach can be criticised on the grounds of validation problems. Rein (96) concedes that 'the validity of the explanation of what happened - interpreting why the sequences of events occurred - is much harder to assess. The validity of explanations is elusive'. All that can be asserted is that 'the story should be the simplest, most comprehensive, internally consistent explanation we can offer, and it should also be consistent with possible explanation of similar events'(97).

RESEARCH SETTING

The two health boards, (hereafter referred to as Alpha and Beta), selected for study were chosen for two principal reasons: (1) they were medium-sized boards, (both in terms of population and in terms of resource allocations), were reasonably representative of the sorts of problems, pressures and constraints facing all fifteen health boards in Scotland and both had a mixture of urban-industrial and rural areas; and (2) the size and structure of the two boards were such that one researcher could cope with their intricacies. Both boards were divided into two districts. Diagram 3 shows, in simplified form, the structure of the Scottish NHS listing the principal

DIAGRAM 3 MAP OF PRINCIPAL DECISION ACTORS IN DEVELOPMENT FUND ALLOCATIONS

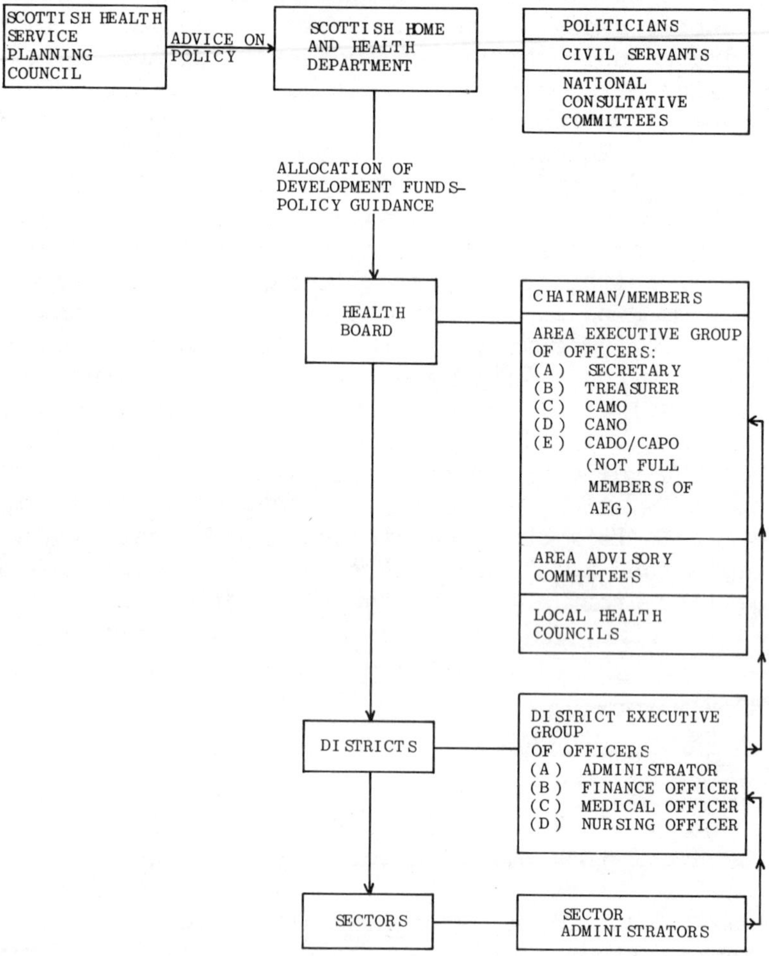

NOTES:

1 There are no advisory committees at district level in Alpha. They are present in Beta.
2 The DEG has a line management relationship to the AEG; sectors are accountable to districts (indicated by arrows in diagram).
3 Local Health Councils tend to operate at district level but they are set up by the area.

decision-makers involved in the decision process observed.

Naturally, each of the fifteen health boards has its own peculiar characteristics, not just those arising from the personalities of members and officers but also those resulting from the facilities provided, and the type and size of hospitals maintained. In these, and other suchlike, respects Alpha and Beta differed, although they were similar in overall terms, as noted. It is not possible, therefore, to pinpoint a typical health board. However, in choosing between 'most similar systems' and 'most dissimilar systems' the former strategy prevailed. It was partly in an attempt to overcome some of the more extreme variations among certain health boards, e.g. the island authorities and the Highland board, all of which have special problems to deal with which are not found elsewhere, that the case study confined its search for appropriate units of analysis to those boards with what might loosely be termed average characteristics, i.e. in terms of population size and funding (see Table 3.1), and which were situated in the mainstream of health problems facing all boards to some extent but especially those in lowland Scotland where population and health care needs are concentrated.

The allocation of development funds (DF) was selected for the following reasons: (1) the decision area was well-defined, was reasonably self-contained with a clear point of entry and definite cut-off point when decisions on allocations had been taken; (2) the funds represented the main (in practice often the only) source of 'new' money received by health boards, and were important if changes were desired, or if deficiencies within the Service required attention; (3) the allocation of DF involved the principal parts of the organisation structure of health boards, since the two tiers (areas and districts), and the main participants within each, required to be consulted about proposed allocation decisions; and (4) the allocation of DF was not a unique once-and-for-all operation but a procedure embarked on annually by all health boards.

A great deal of social science research is conducted in imperfect environments. All decision-making

TABLE 3.1 Health Boards: Approximate Population and Revenue Allocations 1975/76

Health Board	Approximate Population	Final Revenue Allocations*
		£m
Argyll and Clyde	460,200	29,880,000
Ayrshire and Arran	374,400	17,492,000
Borders	99,100	5,834,000
Dumfries and Galloway	143,700	10,536,000
Fife	337,700	19,124,000
Forth Valley	267,000	18,909,000
Grampian	447,900	35,644,000
Greater Glasgow	1,129,400	118,924,000
Highland	178,300	15,659,000
Lanarkshire	563,100	30,398,000
Lothian	758,400	69,433,000
Orkney	17,500	933,000
Shetland	18,400	1,131,000
Tayside	401,200	43,852,000
Western Isles	30,100	1,704,000

*Allocations to Health Boards on revenue account for Hospital Services and Community Health Services in the financial year 1975/76.

Sources: Factsheet, The National Health Service in Scotland, Scottish Information Office, 1976, p.3; Scottish Office Finance Division.

studies, unless they are conducted in a laboratory, (which raises other problems), suffer from one overriding obstacle, namely, the near impossibility of being able to capture all the multifarious elements which comprise any decision process in a complex organisation. In his classic work, Barnard (98) noted:

> 'Not the least of the difficulties of appraising the executive functions or the relative merits of executives lies in the fact that there is little direct opportunity to observe the essential operations of decision. It is a perplexing fact that most executive decisions produce no direct evidence of themselves and that knowledge of them can only be derived from the cumulation of indirect evidence. They must largely be inferred from general results in which they are merely one factor, and from symptomatic indications of roundabout character'.

There are other problems too. For instance, as Hall _et al_ (99) are aware

> 'case studies of policy-making overwhelmingly move towards a conclusion - a point of decision. Yet policy formation is clearly a flow of events and actions over time in which few of the participants will be concerned with that development alone ... The researcher raises it to a special position and thereby artificially removes it from the press of _other_ concurrent, overlapping and competing events'.

A similar point is made by Donnison _et al_ (100) who argue that accounts of administrative processes often make them appear 'deceptively systematic and continuous'. The authors acknowledge that the completion of a task, or the progress of a development, seldom fully occupies the time of those responsible for these matters. The decision process, or development, in which one has an interest

> 'more typically consists of one item towards the end of a crowded committee agenda, a telephone call made the following month, a paragraph in a

memorandum prepared over the weekend dealing mainly with other matters, then a hurried departmental meeting followed by a chance conversation between two people on their way to lunch. Such are the scattered incidents - if the researcher is fortunate enough to trace them - which should be threaded together to produce what the participants may later regard as an unrecognisably coherent story'.

One way of overcoming some of these difficulties is to research a decision process by observation, by the study of documentary evidence and by interviews. Even then the researcher can never quite be sure whether or not he has been able to capture all the relevant factors pertaining to a particular decision. A researcher cannot, in most cases, be present at every informal chat in cars, over coffee/tea/lunch, in corridors, on stairs and so on. It is quite straightforward attending formal meetings but the real difficulties arise over the many informal encounters which inevitably occur in an environment where a few individuals work closely together. The impact of the politics of office geography on decision-making practices should never be underestimated. All one can hope to achieve in these circumstances is a description of decision-making which, although incomplete, is acceptably accurate in its essentials and where the missing pieces do not distort reality to the point at which it becomes invalid. This research has proceeded on the premise that what was captured really happened, but that not all that happened was necessarily captured.

DATA SOURCES

There were four data sources:

- <u>observation</u> of selected committees
- <u>interviews</u> with selected individuals
- <u>analysis</u> of documents relating to the organisation of Alpha and Beta, the allocation of DF, and material on a wider basis relating to the NHS generally
- <u>questionnaire</u> circulated to remaining thirteen health boards to ascertain whether observations obtained from Alpha and Beta were typical, or

atypical, of similar processes in other boards.

(a) <u>Observation</u>

It was arranged that all meetings convened for the purpose of allocating DF would be attended and observed. These meetings took place at four levels in Alpha and Beta: (i) area executive group; (ii) two district executive groups; (iii) professional advisory committees; and (iv) policy and resources committee (proposals then went to full board for ratification which was a formality). At area level, the main participants were: the Secretary, Treasurer, Chief Administrative Medical Officer (CAMO) and Chief Area Nursing Officer (CANO) and these officers collectively formed the AEG. The Chief Administrative Dental Officer (CADO), the Chief Administrative Pharmaceutical Officer (CAPO), one or two other officers and chairpersons of advisory committees (especially the medical one) occasionally had parts to play at AEG gatherings when invited but only within their own spheres of influence (101). At district level, the main participants in the two districts were: the District Administrator (DA), District Finance Officer (DFO), District Medical Officer (DMO) and District Nursing Officer (DNO) and these officers collectively formed the DEG. As with the AEG, one or two other officers, like the District Dental Officer (DDO), attended meetings of the DEG when requested to do so.

The various professional advisory committees also had to be consulted on whether or not they found the proposed allocations of DF satisfactory. Of these committees, three were important: Area Medical Committee, Area Nursing and Midwifery Committee and Area Paramedical Committee. The chief participants were the committee chairpersons. Advisory bodies representing consumer interests, Local Health Councils, were not fully established in the first year of the research (Year 1), while in the second year (Year 2) their influence on resource-allocation decisions was not much in evidence, principally because there were few resources available on which to take decisions, as is explained below.

Finally, proposed allocations were referred to the

policy and resources committee of the board for discussion and approval. Members of the committee had an opportunity to question, change or suggest alternatives. The main participants were the chairman and committee members. The full board played a small, and usually unimportant, part in these deliberations (102).

(b) Interviews

The key participants in the allocation process were interviewed. Interviews were conducted with area and district officers, the chairpersons of the main advisory committees, the chairmen of the two health boards, and board members (103). The interviews all followed a similar pattern and were informal and unstructured with open-ended, rather than fixed-choice, questions. Questions about how personnel in an organisation conceive of their operations, and how routine organisational decisions are made, require a flexible method. Standardised questions would assume that both the respondents and the researcher shared similar information about the organisation and operations of health boards.

An aide memoire was used for each interview which listed the topics and issue-areas it was thought desirable to cover in a particular interview. The majority of interviews were recorded on a cassette recorder and later transcribed. The average length of an interview was one hour but some interviews lasted half an hour, while others lasted over two hours. Follow-up interviews were conducted with many of the officers. These were carried out in Alpha in Year 2 in order to supplement data gathered from that board in Year 1. Second (and sometimes third) interviews were conducted after a specific development had occurred, or in anticipation of a development. This multiple interviewing technique was useful in confirming, or refuting, the views expressed by a particular respondent in an earlier interview.

Most of the interviews were conducted on a one-to-one basis. In a few instances interviews, or 'semi-interviews' (i.e. almost collective group discussions), were held with perhaps two individuals or a group of four or five. These discussions were particularly useful since participants would, on occasion, be required to justify their opinions before others who were also 'insiders'.

Interviews were supplemented with a large number of casual 'chats' over lunch, tea, coffee, in cars, on stairs, over the telephone and so on. Many of these informal exchanges occurred before, or after, meetings and were a particularly rich source of data.

Interviews were also conducted with numerous individuals with knowledge of the NHS, including a number of key civil servants in the SHHD and the Scottish Office. Although the case study was not primarily concerned with the relationship between the Department and the two health boards, the SHHD nevertheless has a significant impact on decision-making at health board level. Resources, including DF, are released by the Department and it can impose certain constraints (not always overtly) on boards. Therefore, the relationship between centre and periphery had some bearing on the issues under observation in the case study. This was more in evidence in Year 2 than in Year 1 (104).

(c) <u>Documents</u>

Many documents were received during the research period; most of them directly concerned Alpha and Beta and the allocation of DF. They included reports on the organisation and structure of the two boards and their departments; financial reviews; all memoranda on DF from AEGs to DEGs, from DEGs to AEGs, from AEGs to advisory committees; from advisory committees to AEGs, from AEGs to health board committees; all papers prepared by the boards which dealt with DF, such as lists of proposed developments; minutes of both boards and their principal committees; and a sample of minutes from other health boards to discover how they had proceeded with the allocation of their DF over the same period.

(d) <u>Questionnaire</u>

At the completion of the case study, when several core themes were emerging quite clearly from the data, a questionnaire was devised and circulated to the other thirteen health boards in Scotland. It did not attempt to be comprehensive in its coverage of health board affairs but was primarily intended as a check on the relevance and reliability of the more detailed findings emerging from the case study. Responses to the questionnaire provided some general indications as to where, and in what ways, the two chosen boards were atypical or conformed to an accepted pattern. Despite attempts to focus the questionnaire on a few selected areas, the resulting document was still rather lengthy with fifty-one questions listed. A total of ten health boards completed the questionnaire.

THE CHANGING FOCUS OF THE RESEARCH

When the research was originally conceived, the aim was to look at the allocation of DF in Alpha over a two-year period, taking in a second health board, Beta, in the second year in order to determine whether Alpha was typical, or atypical, of decision-making processes in this area of resource allocation. At the time of embarking on the field work, this approach seemed eminently feasible. But, as the first financial year (from April to March) progressed (during which time observations were proceeding in Alpha) it became clear that the deteriorating economic climate was going to have an impact on spending levels in the public sector, including the NHS. This duly happened. Quite dramatic reductions in the growth monies available to the NHS were announced and Year 2 turned out to be a rather barren one financially. For Year 2, the allocation of DF (revenue) to health boards was in the region of 1% compared with 3½% in the preceding financial year. Inevitably this unexpected turnabout in the economic situation (there had been no talk of an impending NHS development famine when the research began) had an impact on the shape of the project. It no longer proved possible to repeat the observation of the allocation of DF in Alpha in Year 2, nor to discover how allocations were managed in Beta since both boards received very little in the way of DF. The energies of those involved in both boards were primarily devoted to identifying savings to enable essential developments to be implemented through a 'better' use of existing resources. This strategy, as revealed in an earlier chapter, was one of the aims of reorganisation and was a major reason for the emphasis placed upon an improved managerial capability. Perhaps significantly, it did not feature prominently in the decision-making process until administrators were forced by external events to adopt it.

Although the original schema was upset by these events, the central purpose of the case study remained intact. The study was primarily concerned with priorities and with discovering how these were set through the allocation of DF. The fact that such funds became scarce did not obviate the need for priority-setting to occur. If anything, it meant that the decisions involved were that much tougher. What did change, however, was the environment within which those choices had to be made. Obviously, a changed environment demanded a new response from those entrusted with the task of allocating DF. From a setting where developments were linked solely to the acquisition of DF (year 1), there were moves in Year 2 to discover what scope existed for funding developments from savings or by reallocating resources from 'less important' services to 'high priority' ones. Because of these initiatives, the decision processes observed in Year 2 were less routinised, less orderly and less systematic than they had been in Year 1. Instead, they were somewhat fragmented and disjointed, responding to events, rather than anticipating them, to a greater extent than usual (than in Year 1, for instance). The suddenness of the economic 'crisis', the unexpected severity of cuts in the growth rate of the health service budget, the need for decision-makers to adjust quite rapidly from a commitment to expansion to one of retrenchment, and the adoption of a new approach to developments all illustrated the variety of constraints and fluctuations, both external and internal, to which NHS administrators are subject. In such a shifting, unpredictable environment it is easy to appreciate why planning drift occurs.

The focus of the case study shifted in line with these changes from one of observing how health boards managed in a climate of steady growth to one of observing how two boards confronted the difficulties and challenges unexpectedly thrust upon them. It was possible to witness at first-hand how administrators coped with change in an environment that was already confused and uncertain. Quite apart from the numerous internal pressures to which decision-makers were subject, Year 2 illustrated quite dramatically the susceptibility of the NHS to the vagaries of the wider socio-economic environment.

If incremental theories of decision-making have any validity, then it might be expected that change, if there was any in Year 2, would be marginal despite the rhetoric at the time proclaiming that the 'crisis' created unique opportunities for those eager to introduce long-awaited changes in how resources were allocated to various competing interests. Pursuing this argument, it is alleged that in times of crisis more significant changes and innovations are possible which rely less upon historical precedent. This is because the crisis leads to a dismantling of the existing bureaucratic routines and operating practices and upsets the political balance between different groups within the organisation. An alternative scenario is that decision-makers prefer to 'ride out' a crisis without implementing particularly far-reaching changes in the belief (or hope) that 'normalcy' will return. There is a refusal to believe that a new phase is being entered, one comprising resource shortages, and instead the persistence of a belief that the present cuts are only temporary, a hiccup in the ordinary run of events. These are the sorts of issues which arose in Year 2, but which were far from people's minds in Year 1. The implications arising from them in regard to the allocation of DF are explored in Chapter 6.

As the above discussion shows, the case study had unexpectedly to deal with two contrasting years. In Year 1, Alpha was observed according to plan. In Year 2, Beta was observed and the procedures adopted by the board in Year 1 for allocating its DF were probed retrospectively. Alpha was observed to a lesser extent in Year 2 in part because there was less activity than in Year 1, a consequence of the lack of DF. In Year 1, the questions raised by the allocation process centred on the allocation of DF, the procedures involved and the particular individuals involved. In Year 2, these questions were no longer sufficient nor particularly appropriate. The game had changed and new rules were sought. Questions centred on the scope there was to fund developments in other ways (i.e. without a reliance on 'new' money). There was a concern with better value for money in addition to a concern with how much new money could be obtained from a diminishing allocation. New considerations entered into decision-makers' calculations including possible staff lay-offs, the closure of wards and hospitals, more efficient bed usage, and so forth. Perhaps such matters ought always to have been in the forefront of managers' minds but, if they were, they were not much in evidence in Year 1.

CHAPTER 4

Determination of Policy: Development Fund Allocations Year 1

The purpose of this chapter and the next is to relate the sequence of events, which occurred in the process of allocating DF during the period of observation in Alpha and Beta over two years (see Diagrams 4 and 5). The narrative is a cumulative compilation of the evidence gleaned from both boards, which represents a reasonably typical allocation process for DF. Most of the data are derived from field work undertaken in Alpha, since this board was observed over a longer period and at a time when DF were reasonably plentiful. Data obtained from Beta constitute a check on the findings which emerged from Alpha and provide a picture of how one board coped with a situation where DF were scarce, a central theme of Chapter 5.

An analysis of the description of the allocation process in Years 1 and 2, which seeks to identify the major constraints which faced decision-makers, and the strategies they adopted to make sense of an often unpredictable and incoherent environment are explored in Chapter 6.

DIAGRAM 4 Stages of the Development Fund Allocation Process

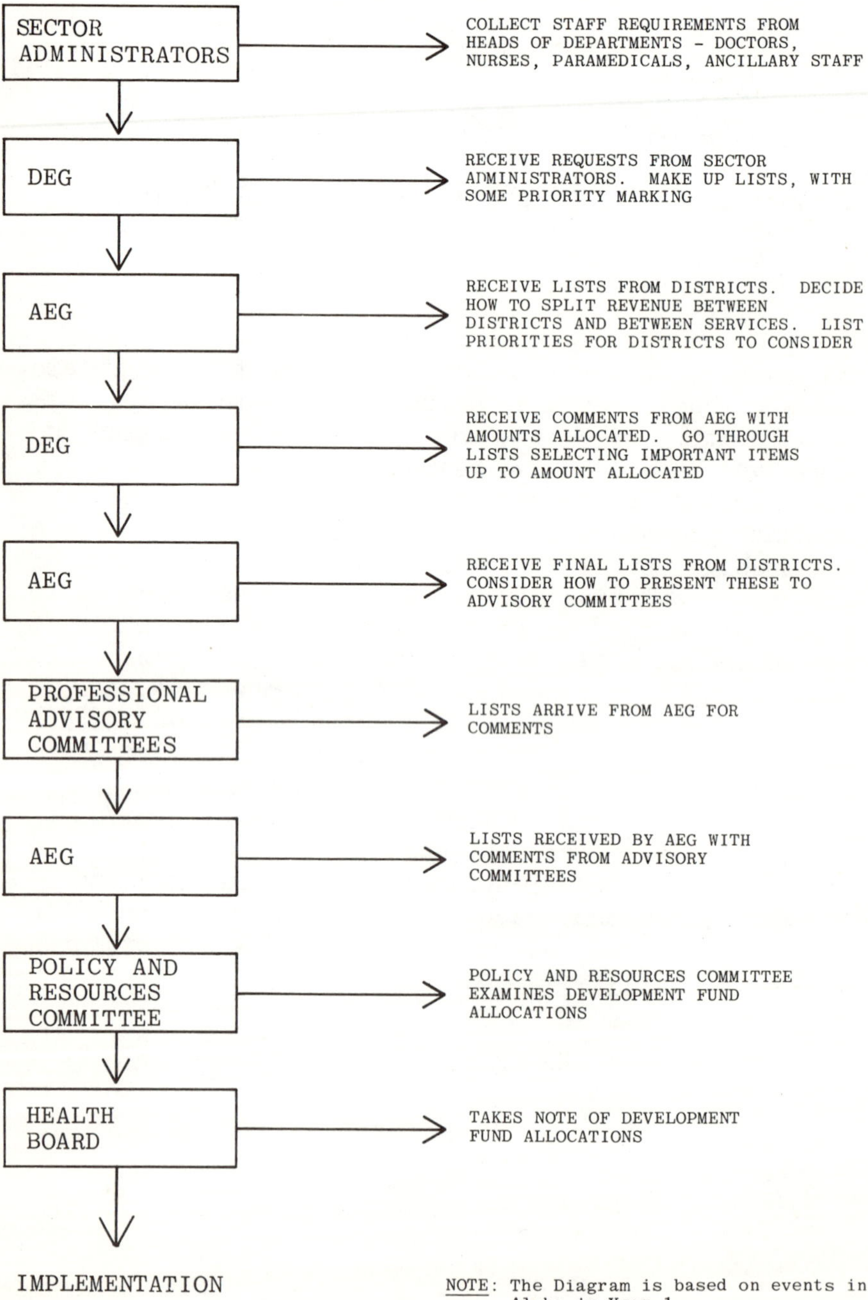

NOTE: The Diagram is based on events in Alpha in Year 1.

DEVELOPMENT LISTS

The allocation process in Year 1 began with the preparation of development lists. In mid-January, the Treasurer (Alpha) sent a memorandum to his district subordinates, the two DFOs, requesting them to submit details of schemes and developments which the districts wished to be considered by the AEG when it allocated available funds. At this time, Alpha did not know what the DF would amount to since the SHHD had still to notify the board of its total allocation for the year. The districts were asked to include on special forms as much detail as possible about each request to assist the AEG in its deliberations. The forms for non-capital developments (which included increases in staffing at hospitals or in the community, and increases in the number of outpatient sessions requiring additional nursing, medical, ancillary and secretarial staff) asked for a description of, and need for, each development in order of priority, the earliest start date for new staff, staff numbers by grade and the full year cost of each development. The lists were to be sent to the Treasurer by the end of the first week in February, which gave the districts around three weeks to comply with the AEG's wishes.

In compiling their lists, both districts referred to their stocks of requests for funds which had been collected over the year; additional requests were sought from sector administrators, heads of departments, consultants and so on. Sometimes approaches by consultants, and others, would be made to the districts direct, or, on occasion, to an area officer who was then obliged to refer the request to the appropriate district officer. All requests made through these channels were added to the list.

Placing the submissions in order of priority was no easy task (see Table 4.1). One DFO (district A), on returning the completed forms, explained in a memo to the Treasurer that:

> 'the DEG considered placing them (i.e. developments) in strict priority order but found it difficult to do so in the short time available and in the absence of both detailed background information and

DIAGRAM 5 Annual Cycle for Allocation of Development Funds

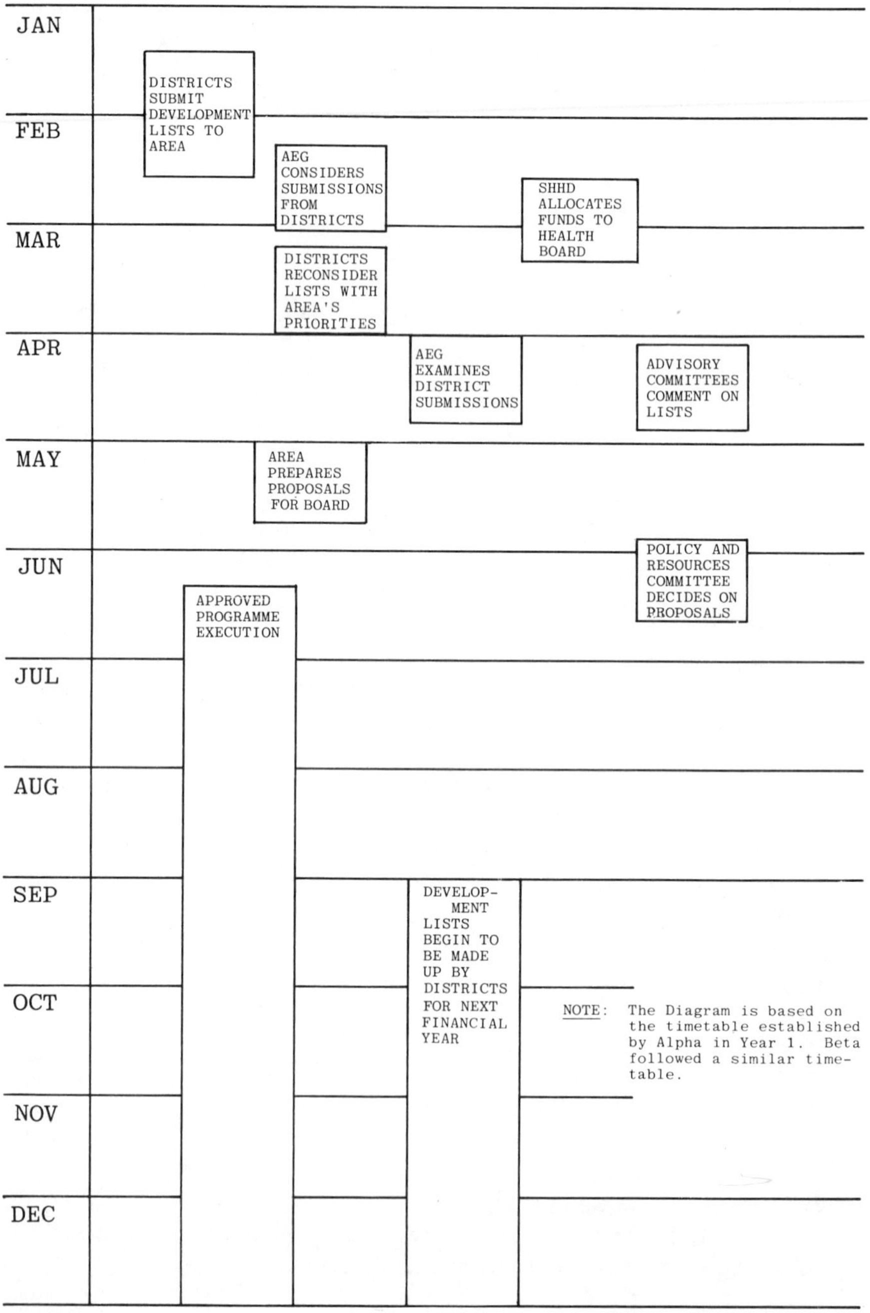

comparative criteria to make an objective evaluation. It was agreed, however, that certain requests deserved to be considered before others and those items marked with an A on the list represent the banding together of our first line priorities without attempting to place them in order of preference'.

Such supporting evidence as was available accompanied the development lists. The other DEG (district B) faced remarkably similar difficulties, although it adopted a slightly different method of placing requests in order of priority. All submissions were considered by the DEG and given a priority rating A,B or C. But, according to the DFO's memo, they 'are not necessarily shown in priority order within each letter'. Moreover, 'due to the short time that was available to complete these forms, it has not been possible to consider each request as fully as one would have wished and also to provide the complete details of the need'. Very little supporting evidence accompanied district B's development lists.

The amount of data submitted to the AEG for consideration was formidable. District A submitted 71 pages of development requests, with each request listed separately. The composition of the requests ranged widely, and included submissions from the hospital service for senior house officers, medical secretaries, technicians, pharmacists, medical records staff, porters/drivers, physiotherapists, domestic staff, etc; from the community service, requests were submitted for chiropodists, physiotherapists, dental technicians, midwives, health visitors, nurses for GP attachments etc. In district A, there were 28 requests for hospital service developments, 21 for community service developments, 19 for the area laboratory service, 2 for developments affecting the whole district, and 1 for the school of midwifery. The requests totalled nearly £405,000 (as it happened, close to the <u>total</u> sum available to Alpha for developments), and of this £220,575 was for community developments, £87,735 for the area laboratory service, £80,035 for the hospital service, £15,650 for district developments and £960 for the midwifery school (totalling £184,380 under 'Hospital' in Table 4.1). Of a total of 71

TABLE 4.1 Developments Lists (Alpha): Total Submissions and Priority Categorisation (Year 1)

1 Total of Submission £820,930

2 Make up of Submissions in Total

	Hospital £	Community £	Total £
District 'A'	184,380	220,575	404,955
District 'B'	258,000	135,875	393,875
Area	16,100	6,000	22,100
	£458,480	£362,450	£820,930

3 Analysis showing total values of priorities in submissions

	Hospital				Community				Total			
	A	B	C	Not Stated	A	B	C	Not Stated	A	B	C	Not Stated
District 'A'	44,405	-	-	139,975	181,065	-	-	39,510	225,470	-	-	179,485
District 'B'	140,800	36,700	28,000	52,500	118,475	9,700	7,700	-	259,275	46,400	35,700	52,500
Area	-	-	-	16,100	-	-	-	6,000	-	-	-	22,100
	185,205	36,700	28,000	208,575	299,540	9,700	7,700	45,510	484,745	46,400	35,700	254,085
Overall Total per 2 above		£458,480				£362,450				£820,930		

Note: District 'B' categorised its priorities in greater detail than district 'A'.

development requests, supporting information was provided for 54 of them (see below).

In district B, the development requests totalled 56, 20 of which were for community services. The remainder, including 3 which were related to the nursing establishment, were for the hospital service. The requests totalled just under £394,000, of which £258,000 was accounted for by hospital developments and £135,875 by community developments. Brief, often general, supporting data accompanied the requests (see below).

From this rudimentary breakdown of the districts' development lists, it can be seen that district A seemed to be placing a higher priority on community services than district B (1). In addition to the districts' requests for DF, the area had also prepared a short list of 8 proposals (this was to grow to 15). These were for area-wide functions and services and included a health education officer, a security officer and 2 registrars. The area requests, at this stage, totalled £22,000 approximately (they stood at £53,000 approximately when the final list was prepared).

As noted above, district A supplied a substantial amount of supporting evidence with its requests, most of which took the form of letters or memos from heads of departments and other senior personnel to district officers or even to area officers. District B submitted supporting evidence of a scanty nature in the form of brief comments which were included on the development request forms. A recurrent theme in most, if not all, of the evidence in support of favoured developments was the pressure on existing staff, whether medical, clerical or whatever, which was (or would shortly be) responsible for a poor standard of service. The arguments deployed to justify increases in staffing invariably revolved around increasing workloads, increasing rates of admission, and an inability to perform essential duties because of diversions to other, often menial, tasks. It was clear from much of the evidence that improved conditions of service for staff (e.g. longer holidays) placed additional strains on the provision of services and were a chief cause of requests for further staff just to provide the same standard of service. In many cases, the supporting evidence consisted of little more than a persuasive letter from a consultant pleading for some relief of his staffing predicament. In a few cases, hard, quantitative data accompanied written pleas. For example, in a request for medical secretaries, statistics showing the rate of overtime worked by medical secretaries in post during a fixed period were included, as were data on inpatient and outpatient statistics over a two-year period in order to show the increasing pressures under which staff worked. Other requests were supported by citing SHHD circulars which laid down staffing norms which health boards were obliged to attain.

Commenting on the overall process of obtaining requests for DF and compiling lists, a District Personnel Officer (DPO) in Alpha believed that it was one which reflected

> 'very much what people asked for. We took what they said at face-value and put it on the list. This procedure had its failings. A lot of correspondence went backwards and forwards and a development was either hardly supported at all or there was little information to back it'.

The CANO in Beta claimed that requests for DF amounted to 'a shopping-list of deficiencies and pressure points. We don't have a long-term goal or direction in which we're going' (2).

THE FUNCTION OF THE AEG

The first meeting of the AEG (Alpha) to decide upon the allocation of DF, in the light of the development lists received from the two districts, took place towards the end of February. Chief officers wanted to allow the maximum time possible for implementation of the developments chosen for funding and this meant determining the allocations quickly. The Group's task at the meeting was to formulate a strategy on how to handle the allocation process and to decide upon the part it would play in this. Most urgent was the need to consider how best to deal with the multifarious submissions for DF in terms of the desired overall direction of services in the area. The meeting was of added significance because it was the first time since reorganisation that the AEG had handled this process. As the Treasurer commented, 'we are all learning as we go along'.

Because the AEG was going through the allocation procedure in regard to DF for the first time, there was perhaps a greater tendency for the four members of the Group to concern themselves with quite fundamental issues like, for example, the role of the AEG vis-a-vis the board, the two districts and the advisory committees. Since the entire procedure lacked precedents (although all the officers could draw on their extensive NHS experience prior to reorganisation, much of which was of direct relevance to the allocation of DF), the Group naturally had to spend time devising an appropriate strategy to enable it to deal with DF.

At this initial meeting, the board's allocation for the financial year was not officially known. However, on the basis of the previous year's allocation, it was possible for the Treasurer to estimate what the DF would amount to. The sum of £421,000 was available for developments and, with total submissions for these funds amounting to nearly £821,000 some potentially awkward choices would be necessary.

In reaching an appropriate strategy for allocating DF, the AEG had to resolve a number of problems. Although these were to some extent technical matters, they had profound policy implications. First, the AEG had to decide whether development monies should be set aside for additional staff under heads of expenditure like medical, nursing, catering etc., or whether monies should be set aside on a functional basis, namely, for particular client groups like the elderly, children, the mentally ill, etc. It was decided that it was not possible at this stage to move to a functional approach. It was envisaged that the programme planning groups (3) which had been established for certain client groups would assist in moving in this direction in subsequent years. More information was required before adopting the functional approach. Moreover, for professional advisory committees it was presumed to be much easier to think subjectively - they were unenthusiastic about a functional approach to development fund allocations. It was far less complicated to look at staffing requirements in terms of additional numbers, for example, six consultants, ten nurses, and so on, without being concerned about the needs of particular client groups.

Second, the AEG had to decide what proportion of DF should be spent on the hospital service and what proportion on community services. The choice was between keeping to the general development rates indicated nationally by the SHHD, and developing one sector (hospital or community) at a faster rate than the other. The AEG decided to conform more or less to the development rates suggested by the Department. National indicators and guidelines would be adopted which, as the AEG members stressed, were only guidelines and not policy statements about desirable developments. Health boards could vary their allocations and were not beholden to a Departmental line.

Third, a related problem, paralleling the division between hospital and community, was the AEG's stance on the emphasis to be given to curative care on the one hand and preventive care on the other. For example, should prevention be given a greater emphasis through allocations of DF than curative services? This was an important decision because it is, in practice, only through DF that a board is able to change direction or shift the emphasis placed on particular services (4). The AEG expressed its hope that at some stage guidance on this matter would be forthcoming from the Planning Council. At this particular time, however, both the Secretary and the CANO were strongly in favour of an expansion of community services. To a large extent, the priority to be accorded community services reflected what was fashionable at national level in terms of the future development of the NHS (5).

In addition to resolving these problems, the AEG spent time at the first meeting trying to define an appropriate role for itself in the process of allocating DF. It was largely a matter of deciding to what extent the Group should become involved in detail, and members were divided on the approach they should adopt. On the one hand, the Secretary and CANO favoured as much delegation as possible to the districts while, on the other hand, the Treasurer and

CANO preferred a more interventionist role for the AEG in the allocation of DF. Eventually a compromise was reached upon which all members were agreed, namely, that although the AEG was not in a position to decide priorities between schemes A, B or C that had been submitted by the districts for consideration by the area, it would issue general guidance on priorities. The main arguments in the discussion are presented here.

It was broadly accepted that the AEG lacked the knowledge necessary to choose between particular developments on other than purely subjective criteria. Furthermore, it was not the task of the AEG to immerse itself in detail but to take a reasonably detached view of service needs and priorities. Nevertheless, there was uncertainty among members of the Group. The Secretary expressed the view that although much in the submissions was desirable, the real question was the extent to which it was practicable. Perhaps unrealistic demands were being made on limited resources but the AEG was not in a position to know whether this was so or not. An example will provide an illustration of the problem. It concerns a request for an improved laboratory service.

The amount requested for developing laboratory services was £90,000. The Treasurer suggested setting aside a sum of £30,000 (i.e. $\frac{1}{3}$ of the amount requested) and it was decided that new posts would have to be funded as the laboratory service wished with the money allocated to it since the AEG was not in a position to decide priorities. A member of the AEG noted that the laboratory service already received £300,000 and wondered whether it was not one of the services that was developing at a faster rate than other services and whether it should be allowed to continue to develop at such a rate. The Treasurer was unsure whether it lay within the AEG's power to stop its development since the laboratory service was not susceptible to the controlling influence of the laboratory technicians. It would be necessary to educate clinicians and persuade them to reduce their demands on the laboratory service before actual expenditure on it could be curbed. Since the AEG was reluctant to continue pouring money into the laboratory service, the Treasurer suggested a compromise, namely, that the laboratory service should receive an allocation of £20,000 although the Secretary favoured a smaller sum. It was agreed to refer the matter to the Area Medical Committee for comment.

This example illustrates three problems with which the AEG had to contend: (1) the inability of the AEG to avoid entering into detailed discussion of particular development requests; (2) the inability of the AEG to become involved in detail in a knowledgeable way when requests were being discussed; and (3) the repercussions that one development could have on other parts of the Service, which imposed quite severe constraints on the AEG's freedom of manoeuvre, i.e. the fact that expansion of the laboratory service had little to do with the service itself, or with those running it, but with the clinical practices of doctors over whom administrators had minimal control.

In its attempts to consider the development lists, the AEG was uncertain how to proceed with the 'carving up of the cake'. So many imponderables surrounded staffing requests. Could staff be obtained, for instance? In some specialties, like geriatrics and the mentally ill, this was doubtful. The Secretary, furthermore, did not think that decisions between various staff requests could be made by the AEG. It was a task for the districts since they possessed (or ought to have) the necessary information which would enable these decisions to be made. The AEG did not know the relative priorities, nor did it know the facts or circumstances behind various requests. The districts, he believed, must be allowed to decide priorities.

There was not unanimous agreement over this course of action. The Treasurer took the view that it was the AEG's job to fund specific developments from the lists and was against giving the districts authority to take these decisions. The AEG should know where the 'shoe is pinching most' and, if it did not, then it was failing in its duty. It was the Group's function to monitor the districts and it was not possible to do this unless the AEG knew what was happening 'on the ground'. At the Treasurer's insistence, therefore, the AEG did attempt to work through the bundles of requests in order to give members of the Group an opportunity to express their preliminary reactions.

This was not an easy task, as preceding paragraphs have suggested.

What worried the Secretary about the AEG's general ignorance was that priority might be given to requests about which something was known to the neglect, or exclusion, of other requests when these might be more important. While he agreed that feedback came from below (i.e. from district officers and others) in one's own field, it was not possible to make comparisons between requests for different staff because one only possessed information relating to one's own sphere of interest, not to the overall scene. The sort of comment the AEG could usefully make to a district would be of the order that, for example, as regards hospitals X and Y a balance was necessary between them to avoid one being favoured over the other. It was, the Secretary agreed, essential for the AEG to be made aware of pressures within the Service, but in attempting to scrutinise individual appointments in detail, it was on riskier ground. In the position the AEG found itself, it could neither be for, nor against, a particular staff appointment. All one would be doing, if one had a particular interest in a specialty, would be making sure that it received preferential treatment. The Secretary doubted whether it was sufficient, in deciding between individual requests, that a mere feeling for a particular appointment should prevail over all else. At the very least, in deciding whether, say, medical secretaries were more important than surgical assistants, information was necessary for this kind of exercise.

It was finally agreed, as already noted, that the AEG would issue general guidance to the districts on the overall provision of services and that it would decide the direction in which the Service as a whole should move. The strategy to be pursued was that DF would be divided between the two districts who would review their current development lists, revise them on the basis of the funds available to them and in the light of the AEG's comments on developments it would like to see given priority, and submit these to the AEG for approval.

The first meeting of the AEG has been dwelt on because it raises several crucial issues. A recurrent theme of the meeting was where the balance ought to lie between direction from the centre (the AEG), and the degree of latitude to be afforded the periphery (the DEGs). A striking observation was the apparent confusion (at a restrained level) within the AEG as to its precise role in the allocation of DF. It was clear from the initial meeting that the AEG's conception of its policy-making role, and its relationship with the two DEGs, remained to be worked out. The various exhortations to be found in the 'Blue Band Circulars' (6) and elsewhere proved to be no substitute for 'muddling through' on the job. The atmosphere within the AEG was one of 'cautious groping' as officers attempted to make the new structure work in a way that was acceptable to everyone even if it was not necessarily in the way that had been intended.

It was interesting to observe at the first meeting the different stances taken by officers. Whereas the Secretary was for allowing the district officers the freedom to spend the DF as they thought best while the AEG maintained an overall balance of services throughout the area, the Treasurer took a more cautious view of the merits of delegation. His concern with finance, budgeting and bookkeeping led him to perceive the AEG's role, to a great extent, as a monitoring and controlling one, which involved keeping the districts' autonomy within well-defined limits.

The second AEG meeting was held about three weeks later. On this occasion, there was less discussion about an appropriate role for the AEG in allocating DF, and much more about how the DF were to be allocated both as between the two districts and the area, and as between the hospital service and the community service. An attempt was also made to establish priorities, or at least to agree on those developments that the AEG considered to be priorities. At this meeting, the involvement of advisory committees and the health board in the allocation process was discussed, and a timetable was fixed for the remainder of the process which was expected to be completed by early summer.

The factor which more than anything else contributed to a concentration of minds at the meeting was pressure of time. It is not being facile to say that the time factor <u>forces</u> decisions to be made, and compromises to be reached, when otherwise there could be no decision or, at any rate, considerable delay. Members of the AEG were concerned that almost half a year would have elapsed before developments approved by the health board would be implemented.

Of the £421,000 available for developments, it was proposed to allocate £67,000 to maintenance, £50,000 to reserve, and £229,000 to priorities within the two districts, some of which were identified by the AEG. Of this figure, £75,000 was to be made available for the hospital service and £154,000 for the community service. This left a balance out of the total sum of £75,000 which was to be used to finance area developments.

It was felt that since one of the districts (district A) was considered to be more affluent in terms of resources and facilities (an imbalance - if it was one - with historical origins) then the 'underprivileged' district (district B) ought to receive a larger injection of funds in order to improve its standard of services. In this way, the AEG would be fulfilling its function of equalising inequalities in the area and of achieving an overall balance of service provision between the two districts. Of the £229,000 or so available for district developments, district B received £100,000 and district A received £130,000.

The summary of priorities, prepared by the Treasurer on the basis of discussion in the AEG at its first meeting and of his knowledge of area priorities for the services it provided, recommended that in district A the bulk of its DF should be spent on priorities in the community service - health visitors and midwives. The bulk of funds going to district B should be spent on hospital developments in the field of mental health (a national priority area). A primary factor in this decision was the location in the district of a 420 bed mental deficiency hospital. Most of the AEG's priorities also lay in the hospital service. The Treasurer stressed that his list of priorities did not necessarily reflect those of the districts. It was agreed at the meeting that if the districts could give good reasons for not complying with area priorities that would be acceptable. If not, the AEG would direct the offending district(s) to implement particular developments.

This still left some difficulties to be resolved in the area/district relationship over the allocation of DF. It was essential that the districts be informed of intended area developments since these could have implications for services operated by the districts. DEGs should be given an opportunity to comment upon area proposals. For instance, if the area proposed a new consultant post this would most certainly have implications for the district in which the consultant would be located, since it would be responsible for providing support staff. Developments of this type are generally unpopular with districts because they involve pre-emptions of their DF by the area for priorities with which they have not been directly involved.

A final timetable for the remaining stages of the allocation process was fixed. The districts were to be given a 'clean slate' and asked to list their priorities from scratch, keeping in mind the funds available to them and the views of the AEG on desirable priority developments. After the districts had revised their lists and arrived at a final set of priorities, the AEG would consider these before submitting them to the advisory committees for comment. If approved, the principal standing committee of the board, the policy and resources committee (PRC), would examine the proposed allocations. In the meantime, a paper would be submitted to the PRC giving details of the DF available. The timetable was designed to enable developments to be implemented as quickly as possible. Of all the advisory committees, the AMC gave the AEG most cause for concern. Officers thought that the AMC might suggest changes in direction different from those proposed. The other advisory committees were not expected to present any problems. Indeed, it was doubted whether the nursing or paramedical committees were sufficiently well organised to tackle the task.

THE DISTRICTS' DILEMMA

In the middle of March, the Secretary (Alpha) sent memos to the two DAs, giving details of the board's revenue allocation for Year 1 and the DF that were available. District A's allocation of £130,000 was to be split as follows: Hospital £68,000 and Community and School Health £62,000. District B, the smaller of the two, was allocated £100,000 to be split as follows: Hospital £52,000 and Community and School Health £48,000. In drawing up spending plans, each district was requested to take note of certain policies which the area favoured for development. The AEG made it clear that it would 'give particular consideration to the implementation of the stated policies in (its) consideration of the submissions'. Also listed in the memos were the priorities which came within the area's responsibility so that the districts would be aware of their existence. Both districts were requested to submit their proposals to the AEG by the end of March.

District A had one meeting to decide upon its final list of allocations, whereas district B took two meetings to complete its business. For both districts, the task of setting priorities was an important one; it was also an almost impossible one. The DEGs had to prune quite drastically their original lists of submissions and since requests in both districts far exceeded the funds available, the exercise was a messy one. Indicative of the near-impossibility of arriving at a set of 'correct' priorities was a comment from one DA: 'We'll (i.e. the DEG) be drawing them (i.e. items on which to spend DF) out of a hat'.

The discussions in district B were more protracted than those in district A. Members of the DEG (district B) were agreed that the developments the AEG had selected for the district to rate as high priorities would have to be included in their final submissions or else the AEG could overrule the DEG. The lists for community developments were examined at the first meeting. Only submissions listed as As were considered; the Bs and Cs were set aside. Not that this made the selection of a final list much easier because, in the case of community developments, there were only 3 Bs and 3 Cs but 22As. The As totalled £114,000 against the £48,000 available for community services.

The DEG proceeded to work through the lists item by item. It was very much a bargaining and a negotiating situation, with members of the DEG competing with one another in order to get what they could for their own services, while, at the same time, striving to reach consensus on the various allocations. Members performed a dual role: (1) as individual officers representing particular interests; and (2) as members of a team trying to decide what was best for the district as a whole. It was not always easy to reconcile the two roles. A few examples of the development requests considered by the DEG will suffice to convey an impression of how the Group operated.

1. Nursing auxiliaries. There was a request for six part-time nursing auxiliaries to enable care to be given to the elderly within their homes. The DNO said this development was important because nurses were under great strain. The DA was in favour of appointing three part-time nursing auxiliaries, believing that these would at least make for an improvement in the service and would be better than nothing. But the DNO held out for six, although this was later reduced to five in order to arrive at the total allocation of £48,000; at this stage in the proceedings, the DNO was not prepared to consider anything less than the number of auxiliaries requested. Her argument was that nursing used to be a case of 'lulls and bursts' but that there were no lulls now. At this point in the meeting the DA was becoming concerned. The Group had only examined five items, most of which had been approved, out of about twenty. At this rate, the £48,000 would soon be gone. He wondered if the nursing auxiliaries had a high priority over other requests (including other nursing ones) and reminded the DNO that GP attachments were still to come. In the DA's view, the DEG seemed to be getting nowhere. Items had to be rated in order of priority. The DFO intervened to point out that by insisting on six part-time auxiliaries at this stage, the DNO was 'wanting her cake and eating it'. The DNO retorted that she was simply aware of the stresses and strains on nurses, a point she repeated several times during the meeting.
2. Health visitors. This was also an area priority for the district. The DNO emphasised that the number of health visitors requested, $7\frac{1}{2}$, were necessary. But the DA's view was that one had to realistic and recognise that this number were not available. If there was no hope of appointing $7\frac{1}{2}$ health visitors,

then there was no point in allocating monies for that number. He suggested that the DEG put in for 2 and raise this number later if staff were available.

3. Enrolled nurses. These were required for GP attachment to improve the quality of service given. The DNO wanted 5 to be recruited and once again, the DA thought this was unrealistic. Nursing was receiving a huge boost with 5 enrolled nurses and 6 part-time nursing auxiliaries. Which were more important? The DNO was of the opinion that enrolled nurses were more valuable. It was pointed out that the district could not allow so much money, from limited resources, to be injected into the nursing establishment. Trimming was necessary in the competition for scarce resources. According to the DA, the trimming that had taken place up to that point had been for reasons which had nothing to do with the necessity or otherwise of particular developments. For example, dental services had been trimmed because of confusion over what the CADO (who attended the DEG meeting in place of the DDO) wanted (see 6 below). The requests for health visitors had been trimmed because the number wanted was unrealistic, given the staff likely to be available. However, if $7\frac{1}{2}$ health visitors had been available, then $7\frac{1}{2}$ would have been recruited. In short, the developments that had been trimmed had been done so for reasons that had much to do with factors other than the exercise of free choice. The DNO was under constant pressure from her colleagues to trim. She responded by repeating her remark about nurses being under strain. By implication, she was refusing to consider strains elsewhere in the service. Finally, in this particular instance, with the DA repeating his dictum that something was better than nothing and was an improvement in the level of service, the DNO settled for 3 enrolled nurses as opposed to 5.

4. Clerical assistance for nursing officers. Over this request for 2 part-time shorthand typists, the DA said a job description was necessary as well as more information. The district had not quantified how the work was to be done; what exactly were extra staff needed for? The district, according to

the DA, 'haven't done enough homework on it yet'. The DNO was forceful on the issue, claiming that she had assessed the need by going round asking nursing officers what their needs were and identifying things that were not being done. Her recommendation that clerical assistance was necessary in the form of 2 shorthand typists (part-time) was based on what the average nursing officer needed. But the rest of the DEG was not convinced of the need. No action was taken.

5. Physiotherapists. Again, the problem of staff availability facilitated trimming. An original request for 2 physiotherapists was reduced to 1. The DA was pleased - in his opinion a 50% improvement on a bid was not bad.
6. Dental services. There was some confusion over developments for dentistry which the CADO was unable to resolve. There were requests for 2 dental officers, 2 dental surgery assistants (DSAs) and 1 hygienist. It was thought within the DEG that the procedure was that dental officers were funded by the area, and DSAs were funded by the district, although there was uncertainty as to whether this was, in fact, so. The CADO was to check on this. In the event, the DEG was unable to earmark sums for either DSAs or a hygienist because DSAs were of no use unless dental officers were appointed, which was an area matter. It was decided, therefore, to allocate dental services an amount which was intended to be for either a hygienist or a DSA (should a dental officer be appointed). The DEG's preference was for the appointment of a dental officer and supporting staff.

After the lists of community developments had been worked through, the total allocation stood at £56,550, £8,550 over the monies available (i.e. £48,000). One way of avoiding further trimming was to mortgage the following year's DF. Since many of the appointments would not be made until late in the year, the £48,000 was thought to be more than adequate. But, just to play safe, the additional £8,000 could be included by mortgaging future development monies. In short, requests totalling £56,550 could be submitted although only £48,000, or less, would actually be spent in

Year 1. Such a strategy would enable all the submissions to be included. But there were risks in anticipating what might happen in Year 2. It was not possible to predict events and it could be that no development money would be available. A further snag was that the board (or, more precisely, the AEG) was likely to follow the old RHB procedure for releasing funds and retain these until staff vacancies had actually been filled by districts. The districts, therefore, would not receive a block allocation but would only be able to draw funds as, and when, necessary. Therefore, the district was not in a position to mortgage Year 2's DF even if it had wished to do so.

A second possibility was to leave requests on the development list but to submit them with lower prices attached. The DA, always anxious to further the district's interests, was convinced that the district could execute such a manoeuvre without being discovered by the area. But the DFO was unenthusiastic about the idea, objecting to the confusion that would result for his staff in their efforts to balance the books. What prompted the DA to suggest such a course of action was the knowledge that the area would probably control the allocation of DF and not the districts. The DA also knew that because the district would be unable to spend £48,000 within the year, the area would transfer the remainder to non-recurring expenditure thus preventing the district from using revenue funds for revenue purposes which it could plan for in advance of the area.

It seemed, then, that the DEG had no alternative but to prune the list of community developments to £48,000. This was achieved after considerable trimming of developments, mainly on the nursing side since there was more scope for reductions under this expenditure head than under others, both because large numbers of nurses had been requested (unlike other staff categories), which meant that they could afford to lose a few (it was easy to make paper reductions in staffing whatever the actual service needs may have been), and because it was usually impossible to fill all vacancies. At the end of the day, of the 22 A-rated requests, 7 developments were not approved, while 12 had been (of which 5 had been altered to arrive at the correct total) plus the 3 area-financed developments.

Hospital developments in district B were discussed at a second meeting the following day. Area priorities for the hospital service were discussed first, one of which led to lengthy discussion. In its original lists, the district had submitted a request for one clothing manager and 9 ward housekeepers at an MD hospital. These developments involved expenditure in the region of £20,000 and the AEG had rated them top priority, in part because of general staff shortages at the hospital (ward housekeepers would relieve nursing staff of non-recurring duties), but also because it was national policy to give priority to long-stay hospitals. However, with only £52,000 to spend on hospital developments, the DEG was reluctant to spend almost half this amount on these two developments. The DFO pondered the possibility of improving the existing nursing situation as an alternative to appointing all these new staff. It was finally agreed that 3 ward housekeepers would be financed from DF while the remainder (i.e. 6), and the clothing manager, would remain on the lists and would be financed from underspending on the nursing budget as had been intended for some time. The DA defended these tactics on the grounds that it was not going to be possible to gain access to DF since, as already noted, these were to be held by the AEG until required for each specific development as it was implemented. Since the districts were unable to control their own allocations it would not be possible to switch funds from one activity to another. Hence, flexibility at district level in funding developments would have to be achieved through devious means if at all.

The saga of these particular developments provides an example of the friction which was present from time to time in the area/district relationship. Not only was the DEG, especially the DA, frustrated at its inability to receive its share of DF and to switch these around as it considered most appropriate, but it had made little headway with its original plan to finance these two developments from underspending in the nursing budget for the MD hospital in question. To do this, approval from the AEG was necessary but none had been received. The DFO commented, 'we never get formal approval, only approval in principle'.

As at the first meeting, only the A-rated requests were examined, although there was a large number of them. Out of a total of 36 hospital developments, 7 were Bs, 7 were Cs while 22 were As. The As totalled £165,800 as against the £16,000 that remained of the original £52,000. Once again, savage pruning was unavoidable. Two examples follow of allocation decisions taken at the meeting.

1. Radiographers. According to the DMO, 2 radiographers were 'desperately needed'. The sum required for these appointments was over £5,000 and there was no problem about availability. While the DMO accepted that the auxiliary head at the hospital where the vacancies were was underspent, this had not necessarily occurred under the radiography head. He explained that the demand for radiographers was the result of a new consultant radiographer who had been appointed at the beginning of the year; before his arrival there had been no demand for additional staff; the consultant had created a demand for this service and now required support staff to cope with the expansion. The DFO thought that perhaps the consultant was not doing more work but rather that others were doing less, but this was not pursued. The DA pointed out that if a consultant was appointed, it was essential to consider any necessary support services that would be required. He maintained that the AEG (which was responsible for senior staff appointments) should consult the districts when consultant posts were filled in order that the DEGs could consider what support services would be required (districts being responsible for providing these services). This was a prime example of the tensions which can occur in a two-tier structure when closely related functions are split between the tiers. Districts were not anxious to fund support services for consultants since these were pre-emptions on their DF, although in the present case, the 2 radiographers were accepted as being necessary (the allocation was reduced to 1 at a later stage of the proceedings - see below). The DNO interjected

to say that she could put forward similar arguments, to those of the DMO's, for more nurses. The DA replied that that was why 'we gave you all the nurses yesterday' (i.e. at the meeting which decided allocations to community developments).

2. Nursing staff (maternity hospital). This development was a late addition. After the lists had been scrutinised, the DA asked if members of the DEG had other requests in the light of changed circumstances since the original lists had been prepared. The DNO raised the matter of additional nursing staff at the maternity hospital although she agreed that the need had not been well-defined and that there were conflicting reports as to the necessity of more nurses. A factor in favour of the development was that the hospital was underspent by £1,700. Against this, the DFO pointed out that the national birth rate was declining. The DA, moreover, was anxious to ascertain what sort of case had been made out for the request. In his view, the increase in staff establishment wanted was too great and, therefore, suspect. Since the development was not ready for funding on the basis of information available, the DEG decided to leave the matter meantime. It had not 'gone through the sieve' (i.e. the DEG). The DA emphasised that before any request went on the development lists, it had to be well-argued and searching questions must be asked within the DEG. A case for a development had to withstand detailed questioning.

Despite the DA's comment, items did, on occasion, appear on development lists without sufficient supporting data (as above).

Of the 22 A-rated developments, 8 were not approved (this rose to 9 after a further cut later in the meeting). One request was rejected on the grounds of insufficient information, and three requests for additional nursing staff 'to bring present establishment up to satisfactory level' were rejected because the establishment figure was unrealistic - there were neither the people nor the funds to fulfil it. Of the 13 remaining A-rated developments, 4 were altered, i.e. a request for 9 ward housekeepers was reduced to 3 (the rest, as mentioned earlier, were to be funded from underspending on the nursing budget at the hospital in question); a request for a clothing manager was also to be financed from underspending on the nursing budget rather than from DF (see above); a request for 2 domestic assistants at one hospital was reduced by half, and a request for 15 domestic assistants, 4 of which were A-rated, at another hospital was also reduced by half, from 4 to 2, on the principle that this was 'better than nothing'. After further 'horse-trading' (the DA's term to describe the activity in which he and his colleagues were engaged), the task was finally accomplished.

Throughout the two meetings of the DEG to consider its development lists, tensions were evident between the DA and the DFO, and between the DNO and the rest of the Group. The DNO saw her task primarily as one of getting what she could for nursing and, even if not always successful, she was always forceful in putting her case. The tensions between the DA and DFO revealed fundamental differences in the approaches of the two officers to decisions on DF, and to the district/area relationship. For the DA, the overriding aim of the DEG was 'to get our hands on the money' in order to 'get it over here'. In his view, the present system slowed up decision-making because it involved having to wait for the AEG to approach the districts with non-recurring monies towards the end of the financial year, anxious to see it spent. The DA advocated a procedure that would short-circuit this laborious, and not especially efficient, system and speed up the decision-making process. But the DFO wanted to play the game by the rules. While not objecting to occasional manoeuvring, he refused to bend the rules to the point of deception. Consequently, he was not prepared to inform the health board that the district had staff at hand to appoint when this was not the case, or that 'extra' staff should be appointed, and then proceed to switch resources allocated for the purpose to other preferred schemes. Although the DFO could have been overruled by his colleagues on the DEG, the difference of opinion between the two officers over tactics was not pushed this far.

District A's DEG met once to decide upon its allocations and agreement was reached with a minimum of delay. Although district B had a higher proportionate share of DF allocated to it, in overall terms district A received a larger allocation since it was the larger of the two districts, having 2,028 hospital beds, 4 health centres and 19 clinics, compared with district B's 1,005 hospital beds, 2 health centres and 15 clinics. In addition, however, district A was, as has been noted, allegedly a better endowed district. Indeed, in the hospital sector, the DEG had difficulty in finding sufficient items on which to spend the DF available to it, a situation which was in sharp contrast to district B's experience. In the event, the DEG favoured switching funds from the hospital to the community sector and sought the AEG's approval for this action.

Although there were few arguments over priorities at the meeting, and despite the fact that the DEG was able successfully to fund all its priorities and, moreover, allocate additional funds to the community services, the DEG was not entirely happy with the method adopted for allocating DF. The DFO thought it would be desirable if, in future years, more background information on proposed developments was obtained.

Both districts submitted their final lists to the AEG on time. In his accompanying memo, the DA in district B pointed out that the posts being recommended in the fields of nursing, domestic staff and junior laboratory technicians were in relation to posts approved, and appointments made, by the former BoM prior to reorganisation, for which no funds had been provided. These posts accounted for a large proportion of the district's pre-emptions. The memo ended with a reminder that despite the proposed developments

> 'this still leaves extensive gaps in the health care services being provided in (this) district, and it would be greatly appreciated if any additional recurring funds could be made available, which would go some way towards the introduction of much needed improvements in the service'.

In a shorter memo, the DA in district A explained that the DEG felt that the developments requested for the community should receive rather more than the sum allotted by the AEG, and that a corresponding reduction in the sum allotted for hospital developments had been made by the DEG.

AEG : ROUND TWO

The AEG met to consider the revised development lists at the beginning of April. This gave chief officers an opportunity to examine what the two districts had decided within the priorities laid down by the AEG. The view was expressed, as it had been on previous occasions, that the AEG ought not to scrutinise the developments proposed by the districts in too much depth. This was the Secretary's preference. The CAMO did not favour such a detached role for the AEG and suggested two criteria by which the Group could judge the lists: (1) the AEG must see to it that the districts did not get out-of-line, that is, they must be kept in balance; and (2) the AEG must see that development proposals were realistic. According to the CAMO, it was the task of the AEG to examine each item, although he accepted that chief officers were not well placed to do so because of a lack of appropriate data. The AEG, however, was prepared to accept the districts' views on proposed developments and the general consensus was that members were 'reasonably happy' with the lists as they stood.

There was discussion at the meeting to decide where a line should be drawn between the area financing staff appointments at senior level, and the districts having to finance supporting staff for these senior appointments. This, as noted earlier, was a problem which rather disfigured relations between area and districts. The matter arose specifically in the light of district B's confusion over its dental services (see above). The AEG decided that a dental officer and supporting staff were to be funded by the health board, rather than the dental officer by the area, and supporting staff by the district concerned. Splitting the provision of services between two tiers was recognised to be far from ideal. The procedure to be adopted would involve the area claiming back from the district the cost of providing supporting staff. However, there remained a problem in deciding upon an appropriate division of responsibilities between area and district in this matter because area appointments had all kinds of ramifications at lower levels. Although it was preferable, as a rule, if the area could finance supporting staff for senior appointments, it was not easy to know where to stop. For example, with new consultants, the area might be expected to appoint new house officers, registrars, nurses and perhaps other staff as well. Moreover, there was an added complication, namely, that the more that was added on to any appointment in the way of supporting staff, the more difficult it was to confirm the appointment since it involved a considerable amount of money. Splitting costs carried the advantage of spreading the load and making it appear that developments were less expensive than they in fact were.

Finally, members of the AEG were conscious of pressure of time. There were still several stages to go through before the DF were actually disbursed. Once the advisory committees had examined the lists they would be returned to the AEG at the end of April. As mentioned, time was important because once the allocations were approved six months usually elapsed before new staff were in post.

PROFESSIONAL ADVISORY COMMITTEES

Towards the middle of April, five area advisory committees were asked by the AEG to express their opinions on the development proposals. The committees were: the Area Medical Advisory Committee, the Area Nursing and Midwifery Committee, the Area Dental Advisory Committee, the Area Pharmaceutical Committee and the Area Paramedical Advisory Committee. Whereas the medical, nursing, paramedical and dental committees had reasonable numbers of proposals to review, the pharmaceutical committee only had two proposals to comment upon.

Of all the committees, only the paramedical one expressed surprise and concern at the way in which the proposals from the AEG had come 'out of the blue'. There was indignation and puzzlement that no approach had been made either to the committee or to any members of it to discover their suggestions for improving services. This was the first occasion on which those attending the meeting had heard about these proposals. In particular, members wanted to know the source of the information cited in support of the proposals, and who had suggested these particular developments and when? In the committee's view, immediate necessities had been taken up by the districts on an arbitrary basis. Not all the proposals were supported with arguments and the committee felt it was wrong to be asked to comment on them. The committee agreed in general that a much better way of conducting the whole process of allocating DF would have been for it to have been asked for recommendations for additional staffing, which was the procedure followed for long-term equipment needs.

There was also some concern among members of the committee at the alleged bias in the lists in favour of community services, although a speech therapist believed that if such a bias was present this was to be welcomed if community services needed, or deserved, extra resources. What the committee members who were uneasy about the bias wanted to establish were the grounds on which it had been decided that community services deserved additional funding. The speech therapist maintained that since the NHS was now an integrated Service there was nothing to suggest that there was any bias. But the chairman (hospital based) argued that a close look at the proposals revealed a strong emphasis on the community service and that none of these developments should be implemented at the expense of the hospital service.

Despite grievances about the handling of the proposals, the committee conceded that it was probably too late to change the lists. Furthermore, members did appreciate the difficulties facing the AEG in allocating DF. Available funds might not be used for the really vital developments since it was recognised that the area had to spend the money which meant, on occasion, using it for available staff rather than on staff who might be urgently required but who were not available. A current shortage of physiotherapists, for example, was due to an inability to fill vacancies, rather than because of lack of resources. Funds had to be spent on what could be obtained rather than always on what was essential.

Significantly, it was believed by many on the committee that some of the problems affecting paramedicals within the NHS were a direct consequence of their weak bargaining position on executive groups at area and district levels. The chiropodist maintained that paramedicals were at a disadvantage vis-a-vis doctors and nurses because they did not have officers to represent their interests either on the AEG or on the two DEGs. Even dentists had a CADO and DDOs who could be quizzed on various matters and put forward the dentists' views. CMSs dealt with the interests of the paramedical professions but they came under the CAMO's authority and lacked status and influence.

To register its disapproval at the way in which the allocations of DF had been handled, each specialty represented at the meeting submitted a list of requirements based on assessments of establishment figures in their respective disciplines. The lists were forwarded to the Secretary along with an accompanying letter from the committee requesting better consultation in future. The committee expressed dismay at the lack of an overall development strategy and wanted to see a more systematic means of assessment evolve.

At the end of April, all the advisory committees had submitted their comments to the AEG. The nursing committee had 'no criticisms of the proposals' to report. Although the proposals had arrived too late for discussion at the committee's April meeting, the chairman had made the information available to members. The pharmaceutical and dental committees also approved of the proposals submitted to them. No official written reply was received from the medical committee but the AEG, through the CAMO who maintained close relations with the committee, was informed that it had no objections to the proposals. The paramedical committee, as mentioned, replied at length. While it 'unanimously agreed to endorse the proposals put forward by the AEG', the committee wanted it to be known that:

> 'in view of the fact that, with the exception of the chiropodists and the two area posts, none of the professions concerned were aware that submissions had been put forward for additional staff, the

committee would be pleased to know where the supporting data put forward on behalf of these proposals emanated from. There appears to have been no attempt, at district level, to approach the paramedical professions concerned and formally request their own comments on establishment figures. If this was the case the paramedical committee wish to voice their disapproval at the way in which information is being collated'.

Replying to the letter, the Secretary wrote that:

'in a number of cases the requests for additional staff have their origins in submissions we inherited from the former BoMs. In other cases the DEG could see the need for additional paramedical staff. One difficulty is, of course, that the paramedical professions have, as yet, no one person at district or area level to represent their interests. The position will, of course, change when we appoint such officers as Area Chiropodist. Nonetheless, it would be unrealistic to expect all the paramedical professions to have district or area officers and one of our main reasons for submitting the proposed allocation of DF to your committee is precisely to enable you to put forward your own submissions. This may not be a completely tidy arrangement but I would say that the chances of the needs of the paramedical professions being overlooked are very slight'.

On the point about establishment figures, the Secretary noted that they were 'very helpful', but added that there was 'nothing to be gained by adopting higher establishment figures when we cannot recruit up to the existing ones'.

POLICY AND RESOURCES COMMITTEE

It was now the turn of board members to have their say on the proposed developments. Up to this point, only officers and professionals had been involved with the allocations, and mainly the former. The board, through its main standing committee, the PRC, had been kept informed all along of the progress being made. The final proposals were presented to the PRC towards the end of May.

The report sent to committee members prior to the meeting set out details of the DF to be allocated, and the views of the five advisory committees, and it listed under six heads the final proposals that had been determined: medical, dental, nursing and midwifery, pharmaceutical, paramedical, and supporting services (including clerical staff, laboratory technicians, ward housekeepers, domestic assistants). The allocations under these heads did not distinguish between hospital and community developments. In the words of the report, 'the beginnings of integration ... are apparent'. Nevertheless, the total allocations between the two sectors were distinguished.

The PRC's task was 'to consider and if appropriate approve the proposed distribution of recurring funds'. The meeting was of potential importance since it was to be the only opportunity afforded board members to state their views on the allocations of DF and, if they so wished, to suggest changes. Consideration of the proposals comprised one item on a full agenda. Present at the meeting were 12 members of the PRC and the 4 members of the AEG.

It was apparent that those members who contributed most to the discussion were anxious to get results (and, preferably, to see them) for money spent and to avoid wasting it (which could be interpreted broadly to include expenditure on items on which there was no immediate visible return). Comments were frequently made to the effect that the Service must be improved and that action on new capital projects must be embarked on speedily. Slippages in capital schemes had to be tolerated but gave rise to considerable frustration.

The Treasurer introduced his report on revenue allocations, pointing out that the development rate in future years would not be as great as in the current year. DF for the following year would be half those now available. The total submissions for DF, explained the Treasurer, had been made up from a variety of sources: former BoM requests, priorities suggested by the health board on previous occasions, and priorities which the AEG considered to be important. These had all been filtered on many occasions and had been approved by the advisory committees. The element of the total DF to be spent on community and hospital services respectively had been stated by the SHHD, although the AEG had tried to ensure that a larger element of funds was directed to community services. The Treasurer explained that DF were used for alleviating pressure areas in staffing, and where services were not being provided to the extent one would have liked.

The Treasurer also commented on a change that had been made to the development proposals following a visit to Alpha by a team from the Scottish Hospital Advisory Service (SHAS). The adjustment concerned the domestic staff situation at a mental hospital in the area (located in district A) and the Treasurer simply stated that the AEG was aware that members might wish to give more emphasis to improving this service. Either it was a coincidence that the Treasurer should have chosen this particular occasion to mention the change, or else the incident illustrates the impact that the SHAS can have on a board's priority-setting behaviour. The Treasurer, in making this announcement, was probably anticipating, and thereby pre-empting, possible reactions from members to the SHAS' visit.

Following the Treasurer's verbal report, there were very few comments from board members. One member wanted to know if workloads had been the criterion for deciding whether or not to develop a service and to expand areas of care. But the matter was not pursued as it might have been since implicit in the question was whether the relief of workloads could only be achieved through advocating 'more of the same'. Another member raised the matter of equipment developments and wondered if these were included in the lists or whether they were a separate concern. The Treasurer explained that equipment came within the category of non-recurring funds and that requests for these would be considered separately. The query demonstrated the ignorance of some members concerning the actual operation of the health service budgetary arrangements.

There was, then, no detailed questioning of officers on the development proposals. Officers were at all times in control. Discussion of wider issues involving health care objectives or service provision for particular client groups was significant by its total absence. Overall, members seemed implicitly to trust the officers to a very great degree and, in the circumstances (7), it was perhaps hard to conceive of it being otherwise.

The recommendations for developments were approved with very little discussion and no opposition. The allocations went through the PRC in about twenty minutes. The Secretary expressed surprise at the lack of discussion. He thought that former BoM members especially would have commented on some of the submissions carried forward from the former BoMs. The Treasurer, however, was less surprised and explained how in the former structure he used to prepare a paper each year for the BoM with all the submissions for DF listed plus a list of developments which the officers considered deserved priority alongside. He no longer did this because in his view it was a waste of time. Board members just received a list of developments which the officers had decided upon, and were not, for instance, given the lists prepared by the districts upon which the AEG based its final proposals (although if any members were to request such information it would probably be supplied). For the Treasurer, the absence of any discussion by members merely confirmed him in his view that the whole concept of health boards was unsatisfactory.

AFTERMATH

Although the case study is not concerned with policy implementation (in this instance the actual spending of DF by the area and districts according to the approved development proposals), this is not to deny the importance of this stage which has received insufficient attention in the literature on policy-making (8). However, it is worth sketching briefly the history of an event that occurred in district B (Alpha) which upset completely the proposed allocation of DF. The significance of this episode in the overall allocation process is considered in Chapter 6. Suffice it at this point to say that it illustrates many of the uncertainties and constraints which were encountered in the decision process affecting DF.

The problem over nursing staff establishments in district B was first noticed during the summer of Year 1, after the health board had approved development allocations for that year. It transpired that in 1974, prior to reorganisation in April of that year, the former BoM had agreed to increases in nursing staff establishments for its hospitals without funds being available to meet the cost. For various reasons, some historical (see below), staff had been recruited in error to fill these additional posts, with the result that in the general and maternity divisions the whole-time equivalents of 26.5 staff had been appointed in excess of available funds. This overspending represented approximately £60,000 annually. There was a similar financial deficiency in the mental deficiency and psychiatry division but it had arisen mainly as a result of acceptable staffing levels never having been fully funded. Therefore, the total financial deficiency amounted to a sum in excess of £100,000.

The situation had only come to light that summer because of the upheaval associated with reorganisation and because of an absence of management information. Over a six month period staffing levels rose sharply, but the trend was not detected earlier because the relevant statistics were not used at that time in the way they were now. The emphasis prior to current practice was on financial returns which involved a time-lag before problems, if any, revealed themselves. Consequently, it was not until after the DF for Year 1 had been allocated that it was discovered that the nursing situation in district B was getting out of hand.

The AEG considered the possibility of meeting the cost of these additional staff from non-recurring funds until the end of the financial year at which time, if the calculated establishment was less than that in post, some 'levelling-down' would take place. In the meantime, it was agreed that the district should be authorised to utilise its DF for Year 1 on a limited basis, that is, only community staff developments and those hospital staff developments regarded as priorities should be implemented immediately. Moreover, this should be done while appreciating that the situation which had been brought to light might warrant a recommendation to the board that it reconsider its earlier decision regarding developments pending the outcome of an assessment of nursing staff requirements in Alpha which was already under way. District A, meanwhile, was permitted to proceed with its developments.

The PRC, at a meeting in early October, agreed that the cost of additional nursing staff in district B should be met during Year 1 from non-recurring funds and not from DF. It agreed also to recommend that the other developments submitted by the district and approved be considered against DF that might be available in Year 2. This move resulted from a decision by the AEG, and approved by the board, to freeze district B's allocation of DF for Year 1 because of overspending. While $\frac{1}{3}$ of the DF was spent by the district on priority developments, the rest was transferred to the nursing head. The area agreed to meet some of the costs incurred by the nursing crisis because a comparison of hospital staffing levels in the two districts showed district B's to be lower. The outcome of all this activity was that most of district B's planned developments never got off the ground.

The crisis over nursing staff establishments arose for two reasons which have been touched on briefly. First, with reorganisation in the offing, the former BoM took, according to the DA in district B:

> 'a wee bit of licence. Before they went out of office, if someone was shouting hard and always wanting something and they knew they didn't have the responsibility for looking after it, they could quite easily say "OK let's improve it now because by the time someone's appointed and it starts to bite it's not going to be in our day"'.

It was the BoM's final act before reorganisation, although it had no funds to implement the new staffing levels it had approved. Second, the problems over the recruitment of nurses have historical origins. Traditionally, recruiting nursing staff has been an extremely complex task and, although there are still problems, they were particularly evident before reorganisation. Former hospital authorities were unable to recruit easily because staff were simply not available, although funds were. This state of affairs conditioned thinking on the subject of nursing staff levels, which led directly to the sort of problem encountered in district B. After reorganisation, which occurred at about the same time as the growth in unemployment, nursing staff were more plentiful, and recruitment was less of a problem (there were still shortages in special areas and in some specialties). Recruitment occurred rapidly, with the attendant risks of overspending, because it was thought that as many nurses as were available should be recruited in case the state of the labour market altered. In short, attitudes, which were essentially of a short-term nature, towards nursing recruitment had not changed in line with actual recruitment patterns, and were a legacy from the past when staff had been scarce. In a situation where nurses were in adequate supply, boards were in a position to choose when to recruit and there was, or ought to have been, less need to fear shortages.

As mentioned, district A was able to proceed with its staffing developments. One change was made to its allocation proposals in response to the visit by the team from SHAS to a mental hospital in the district. The DEG requested permission from the AEG to appoint additional domestic staff immediately in anticipation of the recommendations of the SHAS' report. It was agreed that the district be asked to identify those proposals on its existing lists of developments which, in its opinion, merited a lower priority than the proposed additional domestic staff. It is worth recalling that when the original lists were submitted, district A's included requests for 8 domestic and 1 domestic supervisor for the mental hospital in question, although neither was A-rated. But in the final revised lists, there was no mention of the two requests.

DEVELOPMENTS IN BETA

DF in Beta for Year 1 amounted to almost £348,000 while the requets considered were in excess of £900,000. Therefore, the scale of operation was similar to that in Alpha, just as many of the problems over allocations were akin to those experienced in

Alpha. For example, Beta had severe nurse staffing problems in one of its districts (district X) where there were shortages in two large hospitals, one psychiatric and the other MD (district X had 3,155 hospital beds, 2 health centres and 13 clinics compared with 846 hospital beds, 6 health centres and 7 clinics in district Y). Requests for additional nurses for these hospitals came to £87,000, nearly $\frac{1}{3}$ of available DF. However, because of overspending on the nursing budget in the previous year, district X received very little free DF and most of what was obtained went on nursing. Another problem in Beta was area-wide shortages in community services. In particular, community nursing ratios were lower in Beta than in many other areas. Consequently, improvement of these was given high priority, although it was realised that there might be difficulties in finding trained recruits. The emphasis on nursing led district Y to allocate most of its DF to nursing, both in the community and hospital services.

If minor differences in approach are set aside, Beta allocated its DF in Year 1 in remarkably similar ways to Alpha. The two districts compiled lists; the area scrutinised them and selected its own priorities which the districts were expected to follow; the advisory committees approved the proposals; and, finally, the board approved them. Like Alpha, Beta subsequently experienced difficulties over recruitment in nursing which led to overspending on the nursing budget which, in turn, distorted the implementation of developments.

CHAPTER 5

Determination of Policy: Development Fund Allocations Year 2

In his conclusion to the Financial Review for the year prior to the start of this study, the Treasurer of Alpha confirmed what will have already become clear from the last chapter, that emphasis had been placed by the board on using its limited DF to bolster the Service where this was most needed (1). But a note of caution was sounded, in that while Year 1 might still show a reasonable rate of growth (which it did), all indications suggested that subsequent years' development monies would not allow services to be developed at the same rate. As a result, it would be even more important for the board to look very closely at itself to see whether the resources which it had were being used to the best avail for the benefit of patients. The Treasurer wrote: 'We all must be prepared to take, what in isolation may be unpleasant decisions, so that the Service as a whole may be as efficient as possible both in organisational and financial terms'.

DEVELOPMENT PLATEAU

The Treasurer's concern over the future availability, or rather non-availability, of DF was realised, though not immediately. For most of Year 1, there was no indication that Year 2 would be markedly different. The Secretary (Alpha) was even suggesting ways in which the allocation process for DF might be speeded up and started earlier. It was not until mid-July

(Year 1), when the Secretary of the SHHD sent a letter to health boards outlining the forthcoming cuts in development monies, that administrators knew for certain what lay ahead. Their worst fears were confirmed when, in late February, health boards were notified of their revenue allocations for Year 2 in a letter from the Scottish Office. The announcement was immediately followed by a circular issued by the SHHD, NHS Circular No 1976 (GEN) 16, on the use of resources in the NHS. It was followed a week or so later by a third letter, this time from the SHHD, on the cash limits which were to apply to revenue allocations. Together, these four official documents provided the context in which events in Year 2 concerning DF unfolded.

The first document, the letter from the Secretary of the SHHD, was issued to key personnel in health boards and it noted that between Year 1 and Year 2, the growth of current expenditure would be under 2% (in Year 1 it was around 3%). Therefore, in an effort to keep staffing under strict control, boards were asked to avoid entering into any commitments for Year 2, or future years, which would incur large expenditures.

In late February, boards received their revenue allocations for Year 2. These included an element for development monies (which amounted to 1½%). To conform with the government's policy for controlling public expenditure through the introduction of cash limits, the allocation also included provision for the cost of pay awards which might become effective during the period and for price increases as well (the usual practice was for the SHHD to provide additional funds to cover pay awards and/or price increases as they arose). Boards were expected to ensure that expenditure on hospital and community services did not exceed the allocation.

At about the same time, health board Secretaries received a circular from the SHHD (2), which contained advice of a general nature on keeping all 'existing use of resources under continuous review, in order to ensure that they are being used to the best advantage'. Furthermore, members of staff were requested to appreciate 'that improvements in some sectors of high priority in the service will only be possible if savings are made in others'.

Since salaries and wages account for around 75% of the total cost of health services, the circular emphasised the need to bring staffing under strict control (this had also been the subject of an earlier circular in August, SHHD/DS (75) 144). It stated that, 'new posts should not be created nor vacancies filled in any discipline unless it is clear that the post is needed to enable a specific job of work to be done and that that job has the necessary degree of priority ...'(3). Effective control over staffing was necessary so that overspending on the board's financial allocation could be avoided. The circular singled out administrative and clerical staff for particular attention:

> 'The latest staffing returns indicate that there has been a marked acceleration in the rate of growth of administrative and clerical staff, and the Secretary of State considers that in present circumstances firm action must be taken to stabilise, at their current level, the numbers of this group of staff'(4).

The fourth document referred to above dealt with cash limits. The letter informing boards of their revenue allocations for Year 2 had referred briefly to cash limits and this latest letter, issued in March, included more detail about the factors taken into account in their determination. The letter also reported that up until 1980 current expenditure on hospital and community services was programmed to increase at about 1.4% per annum (almost half the growth rate in Year 1). The cost of all developments, including the costs of running new hospitals and other facilities, would have to be met within the sums available. Unlike previous years there would be no additional sums allocated for such purposes. The letter concluded with a plea to boards to place greater emphasis on achieving the most effective use of available resources and on obtaining savings by improvements in efficiency.

A perusal of a random sample of health board minutes during this period revealed a general picture of stasis. Almost everywhere, available monies would virtually all be taken up by inescapable commitments, particularly for running costs arising from capital schemes which would be completed in Year 2. These pre-emptions would leave very little money available to improve the Service. Moreover, the general view was that it would be prudent to assume that this was not simply a temporary setback, but would continue beyond Year 2. While recognising the unlikelihood of there being much scope for improvements, health boards saw the reductions in growth monies as an opportunity to scrutinise priorities very carefully and to ensure that boards obtained the best use of available resources. Restrictions on DF, it was believed, created a unique opportunity for a comprehensive review of present services, since new developments would require to be funded entirely, or chiefly, from the reallocation of existing resources. For most health boards, unless savings could be achieved in revenue expenditure in order to allow expansion, or development, of services, revenue monies for Year 2 would be insufficient.

Alpha's PRC was informed of these developments and was told that from a likely growth rate of 1½%, just under 1% must be deducted for the running costs of major national capital developments in Scotland (DGHs, etc). It was likely, therefore, that the remaining balance for general growth would amount to no more than 0.8%. In respect of Alpha, it was estimated that the amount involved could be as little as £150,000. Against this figure, potential commitments amounted to £440,000. At this early stage, the PRC was requested simply to note the position and to instruct officers to examine the implications of it and report back.

In Beta, a similar situation obtained. In March, the PRC was informed that a full analysis of the financial situation might reveal that a slightly higher level of developments than the 0.8% previously reported would be possible. However, it was pointed out that if junior doctors' salary increases were implemented, a preliminary estimate of the additional cost to the board being £65,000, this would represent a commitment in respect of developments which could not have been accurately forecast. The funds to finance the award would have to be found from within the board's allocation and would not be forthcoming from the SHHD.

THE SCOPE FOR SAVINGS

For Alpha and Beta, a 'development plateau', for that is what the fall in the level of development monies amounted to, was an unprecedented occurrence. To cope with it, each board adopted a slightly different procedure, although both encountered similar obstacles, and both found it extremely difficult to make a great deal of progress.

In Alpha, the two DEGs, the advisory committees and others were approached by the AEG with a view to obtaining suggestions as to how they would see health care patterns being changed in order to ensure that those items which were of highest priority in the health care of the population were not held back because of lack of finance. The advisory committees were approached at an early stage because their co-operation was vital if savings and/or reallocations were to be secured. In addition to these initiatives, the AEG set up a Constraints in Expenditure Committee to co-ordinate the use of financial and other resources. This was a small committee made up entirely of officers with no board members. It was established to identify small savings and to draw up 'Good Housekeeping' programmes each of which would save the board a few hundred pounds over the year. The Secretary did not hold out any hope for big savings in the short-term; these would only come in the long-term although the possibilities were extremely vague. Moreover, they would be controversial since they would involve closures, change of use and so on. Over such matters, one quickly came up against the entrenched problem of clinical autonomy.

Most of the data relating to events in Year 2 were derived from minutes, reports and interviews. Significantly, it was not possible to observe meetings because, according to the Secretary (Alpha):

> 'there have been no specific discussions on this. It has been piecemeal, with <u>ad hoc</u> items on the AEG agenda. These bits and pieces have been pulled together into papers for the PRC. We've been nibbling at the problem. It's an example of an incremental approach to the subject - <u>there has been no fundamental reappraisal</u>'. (Emphasis added).

This remark on the position at the time indicated a decided shift from the board's earlier stance, when it was being proclaimed that the resource 'crisis' provided a valuable opportunity to undertake a searching review of existing commitments (see above). Although the intention to pursue a non-piecemeal approach to these matters by widening the 'parameters of review' may have been sincere and genuine, the reality was less dramatic than the rhetoric led one to expect.

Alpha's Constraints in Expenditure Committee performed a small, but valuable, role in the attempt to effect savings. It examined various suggestions and proposals put forward by the districts, advisory committees and others for ameliorating the financial position, and a preliminary list of recommendations was submitted to the PRC for consideration in mid-March. The economies considered fell into two categories: short-term, and medium and longer term. Suggestions in the short-term category, it was stated, would be effective within twelve months, and included items of a 'Good Housekeeping' variety, such as: (a) improving the handling of mail by making more use of second class rate; (b) using paper economically; (c) eliminating unnecessary telephone calls during peak periods; (d) controlling prescription costs; and (e) controlling the overuse of laboratory and x-ray services. Altogether, there were 22 items on the short-term list. It was accepted that the various suggestions 'might not achieve immediate financial benefit but are aimed more at stimulating staff involvement in cost saving and cost effectiveness'. It was reckoned that if every member of staff could save £10 a year the total saving would be over £50,000. Clearly, some of the economies would be easier to achieve than others. While the majority relied upon staff co-operation in order to ensure success, (d) and (e), in particular, could be interpreted as unwarranted administrative interference in the clinical sphere which might lead ultimately to an erosion of clinical freedom.

Medium and longer-term economies were expected to be effective beyond twelve months. Suggestions in this category (there were 8 altogether) contained policy implications for the board. For example, in dental care, it was claimed that fluoridation of the water supply would, after an initial capital and revenue cost, reduce the level of dental care necessary because of the adoption of a preventive approach to dental health (5). Other savings in this category could be achieved through change of use, or closure, of underused hospitals or units. For example, at one particular Home with 20 beds there was an occupancy rate as low as 25%, and the cost of running the Home in Year 1 was estimated at £30,000. The Committee's comment was that 'many of the cases arise as a result of social rather than health problems', and its recommendation was to transfer the patients to other units and close the Home. Another suggestion for achieving an optimal use of resources was to maximise the utilisation of beds since this would promote greater efficiency and reduce waiting lists at little or no extra cost. According to the Committee, 'this comes down to ensuring the effective use of resources without any real increased expenditure but rather by relocation and a review of the system to increase efficiency'. There would be no direct financial saving but such a measure would obviate the need for increased expenditure (6).

In Beta, an attempt was made to effect savings through joint AEG/DEG meetings. The theme of the two meetings (one with each district) was 'an attack on inflation' and their purpose was to examine the economic situation as it affected developments in the NHS and to find ways of making savings by reallocating resources. The point was made repeatedly that to improve one part of the Service would mean less of something else, since there were not going to be additional monies. On the other hand, it was acknowledged that savings and/or the reallocation of resources were not easy options. On the contrary, they were riddled with difficulties. A DA at one of the joint meetings raised a crucial point (one that would assume great significance in the ensuing months) which was at the root of the difficulties both health boards encountered in trying to effect changes in resource use. He was concerned that if a district managed to save money this would be allocated elsewhere and disappear from the district's control. If this was the case, what incentive was there for the district to save resources? The Secretary did not consider an incentive necessary since everyone was working in a national health service. The DA replied that this was all very well but that things did not happen like that, 'human nature being what it is'. Clearly, there was no easy solution to the problem other than for a district to remain secretive about any savings it managed to make. In fact, the Secretary said as much when he suggested that if savings were identified, the district could spend them without informing the area. The DA firmly believed that enthusiasm was essential if savings were to be made, otherwise apathy would be the result.

Throughout the observed period of resource constraint in both health boards, the catch-phrase on everyone's lips was that resources 'must be used to the best advantage'. No one, however, was quite sure what this meant, and no definition was proferred. Most officers, like the Secretary in Beta, simply claimed that it was their job as managers to see that resources were used properly and that they were not doing their job if they neglected to do this. By implication, the problem was perceived largely as a technical one, to be solved by management processes and techniques. Values and political judgements, although present, remained at a subconscious level, rarely surfacing in discussions between officers, except to the extent that progress in any one direction was likely to be met with fierce opposition from some quarter or other.

Various proposals aimed at effecting savings were considered in Beta, but each course of action put forward raised difficulties. For instance, in district Y there were two hospitals which were high cost as a result of low bed occupancy. However, stepping up bed usage might ultimately require additional staff; a change of use would incur opposition from clinicians; and ward closures over the summer months were not a cost-free option. The possibility of ward sharing among consultants was considered but there were doubts expressed concerning its feasibility when the majority of consultants had fairly fixed views about their wards and how they wanted them run. It was accepted by officers that very few wards would be closed if resistance was too great but that the attempt had to be made.

Identifying savings was no simple task. As one officer remarked, in many instances it was first necessary to spend money in order to save it. An example of this was the community health service, where an injection of funds might lead eventually to savings through a reduction of demand on the hospital service. There would, however, be no immediate gains from such a course of action. Much the same applied to prevention.

The overall consensus in Alpha and Beta was that the scope for savings was limited (certaintly in the short-run), although the attempt to identify some had to be made if only as a kind of symbolic gesture to show that managers were in control, i.e. were managing. But privately, perhaps occasionally publicly, few officers were sanguine about the outcome of these endeavours. For example, the CANO in Beta did not think that the review of existing resources would reveal much slack:

> 'since a large part of the budget consists of wages and salaries. It's an area which is going to be difficult to save in. I think we have handicapped the area by not allowing the district teams to have the right to reinvest any savings. This is what would motivate them towards savings. I see this as a district function. My colleagues, however, particularly the Secretary and the Treasurer, felt that this was not acceptable. They would wish to reserve the right to direct savings to where the need is greatest. I can understand their thinking but I think the price you pay for that sort of safeguard is a diminution in motivation and you can say goodbye to savings'.

The Secretary in Beta agreed that over savings there was a problem with incentives, but, in his view, it was an area matter to allocate savings and districts should not be encouraged to retain them. Nevertheless, he appreciated that the districts would simply disguise savings 'so we don't hear about it. A small sum can be "cloaked" quite easily'. The Secretary reflected that things might have been different if there had not been any districts. He was no great supporter of the district concept, at least not when applied to a medium-sized board.

The districts in Beta were ambivalent in their attitude to savings. One DFO said:

> 'If we make sizeable savings the area will redeploy because they know the priorities of the area. I know ethically it's right but when you are going to a department (to request savings) an incentive is necessary ...'

The DA in the adjoining district thought that the AEG's policy could mean that 'savings are effected but not divulged'. He saw it 'having a deleterious effect over the whole range of functional management' because

> 'I think it would be inherent in anybody to protect their own management area. If I am a domestic manager, for example, and I can see savings accruing in the domestic services, having already made an application to the DEG for an increase in staff to augment domestic services elsewhere, then what's going to happen? The only protection we've got is through the finance department where engagement forms are scrutinised. The finance officer is going to be the person who will act as arbiter. I feel it's my duty to know about savings, but unfortunately I'm sympathetic towards the heads of departments. If a district building officer can save a labourer and he wants a joiner, then is he going to go all out to save his labourer under the area's approach to savings? I'd like to see the functional managers being rewarded for savings'.

The DA, however, appreciated the dilemma in which he found himself. For example, he was able to see that

> 'if the physiotherapists are short, or if a chiropodist or a health visitor is needed in the community and we haven't got money for them, if we can save on a labourer or a domestic the money released could perhaps be better utilised in the community. I can see from my point of view that I

would be managing better if I was to direct the savings towards these community developments'.

Part of the problem, as the DA saw it, was the necessity for the district to put its recommendations, with an explanation of how they were to be financed, to the area.

'When you've got another tier who might say that a district nurse in district Y is the priority, then I begin to get even more sympathetic towards my own district. It's cold comfort to save within your own sphere and be commended on the saving but not to get any betterment of that saving within your own sphere. If I can see savings accrue, as a manager I should be hard-hearted enough to say to that functional manager, 'look, you've made the saving but there's a crying need for a dental surgeon in district Y. I think that's where the money should go'. I can see the global picture but I think functional managers must be self-centred. They're trying to improve efficiency and are getting no reward. As a manager I don't want to be selfish - I just want to get the best for this district. But then I'm not the total authority'.

The Secretary in Alpha was also aware of the incentive problem and savings.

'By and large we've left the districts to get on with their own budgets, (But) I think we'd be a bit concerned if, say, a DEG saved over £20,000 and then used it to develop a service. This situation hasn't arisen yet but I think we'd have to look at it. Developments of the service through additional staffing require area approval. I think we may wish to get more closely involved if only because if we don't there's this danger - that we're saying to the AMC and others that we don't mind doing A, B, C and D, but then if a district goes and does something quite different, somebody will say something. It is area policy that matters, not district (policy). There are two incompatible things here. One might say, on the one hand, that the area knows the overall situation best of all and for that reason we should feel free to decide that if one district makes savings, the most urgent situation might be something in the other district; on the other hand, there's the point about having a carrot. I'm not sure how you reconcile these'.

Apart from the dilemma over incentives, which reflected itself in an ambivalent attitude on the part of those responsible for managing health services, there were other obstacles to achieving savings which the ready availability of development monies over the years had tended to disguise. As the DA (Beta) in district Y put it:

'up to this year we've all got so used to having this percentage development allocation - we've sat back, seen how much it is and then it's back to this business of a little to him and little to that. This is psychologically bad. There's no incentive to examine the existing pattern of work; no incentive to save. (The) new situation might lead us to try and make better use of our existing resources. In this district we've reorganised our vehicle maintenance arrangements (which) will save up to £4,000 per annum'.

The CANO in Beta shared these observations, commenting that:

'development monies have hitherto been easier to come by than better bed occupancy. This is something we've started wrestling with (but) not particularly successfully up until now because as soon as you start querying bed occupancy figures you're thrown back on the medical right to dictate treatment. The only way one can hope to do anything very quickly there is through building up good informal relationships with the AMC and persuading them to sit in judgement. I can't see them doing that very readily. We've got hospitals running at 40% bed occupancy which is an absurdity. It's very difficult to gain medical agreement to discussing such things. We've reached that inasmuch as the AMC chairman has agreed that this is a function the AMC should undertake. I can't say I'm optimistic about any big results in terms of savings. I think that there are other ways of getting hold of money for developments, including this important one of looking at how we're using existing beds, nursing time, etc. I see it as a long-term project rather than as something which will help us out in our present economic difficulties'.

The Treasurer in Beta expanded on some of these points. With respect to those parts of the Service which are underfinanced, for example, mental deficiency and geriatrics, 'the position cannot be changed without developments, whether they be nationally financed schemes or developments decided by the board'. Although the amounts saved by both districts were worthwhile, they were not large in terms of what the board was accustomed to for developments. The problem was that for a proportion of total occupancy bed days of, say, 25% in general hospitals, 50% of expenditure (i.e. half the total hospital running costs) had been incurred. At the opposite end of the spectrum were the MD hospitals with a proportion of total occupied bed days of 37% which consumed almost 20% of the total hospital running costs. The position was slightly better for psychiatric hospitals (27% bed occupancy as against 18.7% of expenditure) and better still for convalescent hospitals and geriatric hospitals, although none of these services fared as well as general, acute services. The Treasurer confirmed that:

'the thinking nowadays is that this imbalance will need to be rectified. There is no immediate solution to this. It can only be a gradual process as monies become available. We now come to the general situation of priorities. This type of examination of expenditure relative to use of resources highlights, or should help to highlight, how you're going to develop your priorities. The mental health field warrants special preference as well as the geriatric field. These parts have been traditionally under-financed compared to the acute side of the Service. One would get into difficulty if one said, 'Well let's move across resources from the acute field to the long-term field'. How

> politically acceptable would that be if you were radically cutting down staffing and the service in hospitals X and Y with a view to providing a better service in hospital Z?'

To achieve a dramatic reallocation of resources was not, in the Treasurer's opinion, within the bounds of reality - it would not be acceptable to the population as a whole, let alone the professions involved.

It is frequently alleged that many of the problems over change, or more rational resource-use, stem from 'technical' deficiencies such as lack of information, or the existence of the wrong kind of information. While there may be information gaps, the CANO in Beta did not perceive these as major obstacles to change.

> 'The CSA and the Department have been churning out bed occupancy figures for many years. The medical profession receives them; some of them they receive and we don't, not even the CAMO. They're put in a drawer or the wastepaper basket and that's it. There's an unwillingness to use such information. It gets back to medical power based on the theory that the medical profession works in isolation. It's a political/professional problem rather than a technical one of lack of information'.

If one were to argue that the problems presented by available information, like bed occupancy rates, were technical in character, then one might also argue that such data were of the wrong kind. That is, one could argue that information is deficient if it fails to engage people's interests in ways they think (or can be brought to think) are relevant. Hence bed occupancy figures are figures churned out for routine administrative/monitoring purposes, and doctors are unable to see how such figures can help them gain insights into the nature, or context, of the effects of their work. Yet, the CANO's remarks suggest another interpretation, one which was considered in Chapter 3 where the view that incremental decision-making was the outcome of poor information, or the wrong kind of information, was questioned. This could well be the case in particular areas (7), but what this perspective has tended to overlook is the political and organisational environment in which information is used. Information is power and will be employed, or ignored, depending on who stands to benefit from its use, and who stands to lose. In the specific example of bed occupancy figures, for many specialties these might suggest that action was needed to improve performance, or to adopt new working practices. Many doctors, understandably in view of their background and training, see information which carries with it these sorts of policy implications as a management tool designed to weaken their autonomy as individual operators. It is, if you like, a further example of the manager's conception of 'rationality' (i.e. what is best for the organisation as a whole) versus the clinician's conception of 'rationality' (i.e. what is best for the patient, and the doctor's ability to practice his skill). This is not to imply that progress towards a 'middle way' is unattainable, but merely to stress that the availability, and quality, of the 'right' kind of information will not, by themselves, be sufficient. The existence of administrative politics must be recognised as an important factor in how information is selected and used in any given situation.

If any scope existed for savings and/or reallocating resources, it lay in the hospital service. Community health services offered no scope because, according to the CANO in Beta:

> 'the resources already deployed there are less. The health visitor and district nurse ratios are fairly low in this area, and we have inherited problems in relation to them. So there's very little room for saving. Anything that's saved in the community requires to be redeployed there. The community will remain at a standstill over the next few years unless we see that as being the priority with what little monies we get. But then our priorities have, in a sense, been decided for us inasmuch as the sum we will be getting is very small. We're already committed by previous BoMs to developments which we'll have to attend to. Last year the developments were spent for us by board overspending. This year they will be spent for us (we haven't enough money to do it I don't think, but they would have been

spent for us) by the opening of two converted huts which are the orthopaedic surgical unit, the plans for which were passed and the whole thing under way before 1 April 1974. So the bulk of our development monies (at least 50%) will be, or would have been, committed to this project.*

The CANO in Alpha suggested reasons why savings were difficult to realise even in situations where one might expect to find them.

'We've just introduced ward hostesses in hospital X and they're doing work which was previously done by nurses. You would think right away that you could reduce your nursing, and give that money to ward hostesses. In actual fact, we don't think we could do this at all because we thought there were not enough nurses at hospital X. The development (i.e. the introduction of ward hostesses) has helped the nursing situation, but it hasn't given them too many nurses. Now this may be because the health board has different standards from the old BoM, or it may be they've got more money to spend, or they've allocated more money to hospital X than the old Bo M did. It's very hard to get a saving introduced'.

Another example concerned sterilising centres:

'The nurses used to stretch gauze, make the gauze, and do all the sterilising. You would think that because they are getting dressing packs they should be able to economise on nurses' time. (But) you never see any saving of any great proportions, that is, to the extent that nurses are standing around doing nothing. They are perhaps talking more to patients. It's very hard to shift the money. On paper it looks good but it's not so easy in practice'.

---

* Funds did become available for this development. See below

This brief discussion of the scope for savings in Alpha and Beta, and the obstacles encountered, may be summed up in the words of a DA in Alpha.

> 'Although people say there are savings ... unless at the end of the day you can reduce your staffing it's not an actual saving. Strictly speaking, there is no reason why we shouldn't look at any service and ascertain whether or not it is effective. If it's not effective then it's the responsibility of management to do something about it. It's not always possible because we're in a social, political climate'.

By 'social, political climate', the DA was referring to (1) the existence within the NHS of numerous professional groups, in particular clinicians, who did not always share the administrators' commitment to rationalising existing services and who, therefore, had to be persuaded of the benefits of doing so; (2) the need for officers to respond, at times quite rapidly, to ever-changing political moods which emanated both from below (e.g. the public) and above (e.g. circulars from the SHHD), examples being the national emphasis on community care, and the requirement to freeze management appointments in an effort to contain administrative costs; and (3) the difficulties in effecting savings, particularly where incentives were lacking and there was conflict, usually latent, between area objectives and district objectives. Some of these themes are returned to in Chapter 6.

THE WAY AHEAD

In addition to the official documents dealing with constraints in expenditure, one other official document helped to shape the decisions that were taken in Year 2 on developments. In April, the SHHD published a memorandum (8) on priorities in the health service for the next four years. Its purpose was to provide a loose framework, or set of guidelines, to assist health boards with their resource-allocation tasks.

The document represented an innovation for the SHHD,

for, as an Undersecretary of the Department explained, the SHHD tended, on the whole, to react to events and pressures of a political nature, and did not operate within a strategic plan for the NHS. The memorandum was a step in this direction, although even this step was itself the outcome of political pressure being applied because of resource constraints. However, it was the first document to deal with the NHS in a comprehensive way. Other policy documents had concentrated on specific services.

The memorandum identified five priority areas: (1) the promotion of health care in the community through the improvement of primary care services and community health services; (2) the development of health services for families in areas of multiple deprivation; (3) a lessening of the growth rate of the acute sector of the hospital service; (4) the continuation of improvements in hospital and community health services for the elderly, the mentally ill, the mentally handicapped and the physically handicapped; and (5) the encouragement of preventive measures. The appearance of the memorandum at this time was a direct result of the 'serious economic situation' which had necessitated reductions in the NHS growth rate, and the document was perceptive in its recognition that the availability of DF had 'removed the stimulus to make a comprehensive appraisal of priorities across all the various sectors ... One effect of the present economic situation is to make the necessity for such an appraisal more explicit'(9). This view, as mentioned above, was shared by many officers in Alpha and Beta, at least in theory. The memorandum pointed out that 'if there is to be any marked progress in one sector it can only be achieved by securing economies elsewhere' (10). The opportunity for rationalisation lay, as noted already, 'mainly, though not exclusively, in the hospital field, particularly in the acute and maternity services, which account for some 40% of the total Health Service expenditure' (11). The memorandum stressed that it was not the Department's intention 'to impose a uniform pattern of development regardless of local circumstances'(12), a strategy in line with the Department's perception of its relationship with health boards (13). But the Secretary of Alpha regarded the memorandum as more than simply an advisory document (or one merely 'setting the emphasis', as a senior civil servant expressed it).

'There are things in the document such as, 'the Secretary of State expects the boards to do something'. To my mind that's very close to an instruction. I'm not saying that one must follow it exactly because every area will look at its own special needs. At the end of the day the Department can exercise a strong controlling role. If anyone wants to go along a road different from the ones outlined in The Way Ahead, they've got to be really justified'.

Not surprisingly, perhaps, the memorandum did not reveal anything to officers that they did not already know. The Secretary (Alpha) thought that it was not so much saying anything new as 'making things explicit'. Officers in both boards were aware of the difficulties in pursuing the recommendations in the memorandum. The Secretary of Alpha explained that one problem with building up the preventive and community services was that boards did not possess control over GPs. Although he was hopeful that the development of health centres would make practice more attractive in particular areas, the fears of many doctors over entering health centres and giving up their own practices had to be overcome before real progress could be made. Another problem, which the Secretary was aware of, was that building up general practice through a health centre programme would not necessarily make for less work for hospitals. On the contrary, 'it might generate more work for hospitals because more referrals may result from such an expansion'. Therefore, the SHHD must be careful not to delude themselves that improved primary care services would in all cases relieve the pressure on the hospital service. The paradox that measures ostensibly advocated to reduce costs, or, at the very least, to contain them, might in fact have the opposite effect and actually increase costs also extended to the measures being considered in both boards to effect savings (14).

The memorandum posed other problems for boards. Most significant, perhaps, was its emphasis on the need for improvements in the 'Cinderella' sectors and in the community health services, an objective which, to some extent, clashed with the Department's concern over increasing staff levels. It was pointed out in the last section, on savings, that a vital area in any attempt to control health service spending is staffing. As a direct consequence of measures aimed at controlling staffing developments, those projects with no, or very few, recurring revenue costs were favoured over-and-above projects with large recurring revenue costs, regardless of what the particular projects were trying to achieve. But there was a conflict between this policy aim and the equally important one of improving community services. Long-stay services would suffer, too, unless there were centrally financed schemes which would bring with them additional funds for running costs (these funds were only available with centrally financed schemes, not with a board's ordinary building programme for more modest schemes).

Both long-stay services and community services could only be dramatically improved with additional staff. The Treasurer in Alpha confirmed that the constraints in staff recruitment adversely affected community services which were labour-intensive. The only institutional facilities in this sector capable of bringing with them additional development monies were health centres. But financing arrangements for these changed in 1975. Up until then, special allocations had been made for health centres. Now, however, they were to be included in the national programme or the ordinary capital programme as appropriate. This change in policy had consequences for Beta, as the CAMO pointed out. It could mean that

> 'only big hospitals or institutions will bring extra money to run something new. Health centre X, which we inherited, was centrally financed but we had to find the funds to operate it. There was no additional allocation. (For community services) you're dependent on the present system of allocation by capitation (i.e. annual DF)'.

The dilemma was that while an emphasis was placed upon the improvement of community and long-stay services, the resource situation made it extremely difficult to do very much about achieving this objective, despite the exhortations of the memorandum. Moreover, as the last section on savings clearly showed, the obstacles to switching large amounts (which, had this been possible, should have greatly benefited the priority areas) were formidable. Consequently, the situation of 'low growth', while widely heralded as an opportunity to reappraise priorities and to shift the direction of health services towards community care and away from excessive hospitalisation, in fact worked in such a way as to contribute to the very imbalance it was aimed at correcting! Of course, this contradictory policy stance was unintentional, being the outcome of conflicting political aims, but it was, in the circumstances, inevitable. It is not possible to operate concurrently two irreconcilable policy objectives without <u>policy stress</u> developing.

Many board members found the memorandum useful, perhaps more than many officers did, since it offered them a set of guidelines by which they could measure the progress of their own policies (15). For instance, the Chairman of Beta had been troubled for some time that board members were not really formulating policy at all. In large part, this was due to the board's commitment to inherited projects.

> 'There was not the money nor the occasion for us to start looking at what we could do ourselves. Now within the last three months, mainly as a result of the Secretary of State's memorandum we were asked to look at our priorities in the medium-term and we spent $1\frac{1}{2}$ days doing that. We decided, in line with the (memorandum's) wishes, to develop the long-term care aspects of the health service and the board is now laying down broad principles on what we'd like to do and what we'd like to see. It's up to the officers to implement these in due course. Prior to <u>The Way Ahead</u> we had tended to accept what had gone previously. The memorandum triggered us off'.

Board members seemed unaware of the possible contradictions within the memorandum (examined above) and were by no means dismissive of it in the way some of the officers were. But then, board members looking for something to grasp which would give substance to their role were not likely to be easily put off. Officers were more aware of the intricacies of the problems which the memorandum set out to tackle, and the fact that the document treated the problems in general terms rendered it less useful to them.

DEVELOPMENT FUNDS - ALLOCATION PROCESS

Despite resource constraints, both Alpha and Beta received small amounts to allocate on new developments. The amounts would have been larger but for the pre-emption of the bulk of available DF as a result of two national policy decisions: the extension of the Family Planning Service in hospitals to include contraception, vasectomy and female sterilisation which had not been provided before except on medical grounds, and the implementation of the junior doctors' pay award. Health boards had no control over these decisions and were statutorily bound to implement them as agents of the Secretary of State. Neither of the pre-emptions was popular with officers or board members who, naturally, resented their inability to decide their own priorities with the monies available. The Secretary of Alpha hoped that in future not so much of the growth rate would be pre-empted in this way. He explained how:

> 'pay awards have historically been funded by the Department. The Department claims that the junior doctors' pay award is self-financing. This is not so. What's happened is that every board has had to use up half or more of its DF to pay for it'.

After various pre-emptions arising from the national policy decisions and from developments authorised in Year 1, Beta was left with £104,000, of which £54,000 was allocated to the development of an orthopaedic surgical unit at an infirmary located in district X (this development is referred to hereafter as Ward Z). The AEG had long been anxious to tackle the problem of long waiting lists for orthopaedic surgery which was why this development was given top priority. The sum of £54,000 for Ward Z was just over half of the total figure requested by district X in respect of opening the entire ward. Beta had a sum of £50,000 remaining for disbursement and the AEG had to decide whether this should be allocated to the orthopaedic unit, or whether it should be put 'up for grabs'. The case in favour of allocating the funds to Ward Z was a powerful one since, from the start, the development had been the board's first priority. The remaining DF would enable the entire unit to become operations. The Chairman of the AMC (present throughout the AEG meeting at which the matter was considered) firmly supported this course of action. Since the board now had Ward Z, his preference was for making a good job of the unit by opening it completely. The members of the AEG shared his view, although the CANO added a proviso that before he could agree to the allocation of DF the practice of having extra beds in existing wards must cease since it was placing a strain on nurses who were unable to provide adequate cover for the beds. Once Ward Z became fully operational there would be no need for this practice to continue. The Chairman of the AMC assured the CANO that the matter would receive attention.

Opposition to the proposed allocation came from the CADO, who was concerned that nothing was being done for dentistry. He was against the £50,000 going entirely to Ward Z when there were problems outwith the unit and the medical profession. In the CADO's opinion, the DF should be put 'up for grabs', and, in this way, the dental service might be able to lay its hands on a portion of the funds. The CADO maintained that the AEG attached insufficient importance to dental care. Members of the Group proceeded to impress upon the CADO that dentistry was not unique in suffering from deficiencies. The CAMO said that they could all produce great lists of staffing requirements, while the Chairman of the AMC went so far as to suggest that no one died from a dental condition whereas he observed patients dying daily from lack of resources. The CADO questioned whether death should be the sole criterion governing resource-allocation decisions. The CAMO advised the CADO that he should correct any deficiencies within his own resources as indicated in <u>The Way Ahead</u>, to which the CADO responded by saying that this was impossible, since one could not reallocate to a non-existent service; in any case, the memorandum argued for more resources to be directed towards the community and away from the hospital service. It did not appear to the CADO that the AEG was following these guidelines. He claimed that

> 'other disciplines (besides dentistry) have problems because of a historical legacy, but not to the same extent as dentistry. If two men pay income tax, one on £1,000 per annum and the other on £10,000, if the man with £10,000 loses £2,000 because he has a 10% cut, that's inconvenient but he's still got £8,000. But if the man with £1,000 loses £200, he has only £800 to live off. That's the picture for dentistry'.

An impasse had been reached between the AEG on the one hand, and the CADO on the other. To settle the matter, the Secretary took a vote, from which the CADO was excluded since he was not a member of the Group, to determine how the DF should be spent. The AEG voted unanimously in favour of going ahead with the development of Ward Z. After the meeting, the Secretary agreed that this decision went against the advice contained in The Way Ahead, although, in fact, the decision to proceed with the development had effectively been taken four months previously, i.e. well before the memorandum was published. Furthermore, there was, as mentioned, an acute shortage of orthopaedic beds with long waiting-lists for treatment. A report (16), completed by a working party of board members and officers in January of Year 2, was not complimentary about the state of orthopaedic surgery in Beta. According to the report, it was clear from the statistics relating to bed occupancy and waiting times that the position regarding delays in the treatment of inpatients in this field was unsatisfactory, and, furthermore, that the primary cause was a shortage in the number of beds available for the specialty. Although this finding was probably one of the factors which led officers to allocate all available free DF in Year 2 to the Ward Z project, it is perhaps significant to note in this context that the report did not advocate this line of action as the *only* solution to increasing pressures. It noted that although the total number of beds available was insufficient, the factor which caused the shortage to arise most acutely was the occupation of many orthopaedic beds for long periods by geriatric patients who no longer required orthopaedic surgery or care of this kind. The working party felt that if such patients could be transferred to geriatric accommodation (the ability to ease transfers between the hospital and community sectors being a primary aim of an integrated health service), the unsatisfactory position regarding the waiting time for orthopaedic surgery would be alleviated. In the event, the working party's advice was not followed, one reason no doubt being that geriatric patients no longer in need of general medical services could not be discharged because of a lack of suitable alternative facilities either in the hospital or in the community. To a great extent, the solution of this problem depended on the success of inter-agency co-operation between health and local authorities which was not well developed in Beta (nor in Alpha for that matter).

Despite the working party's report with its alternative policy option to the one pursued by the board, the Secretary was anxious to stress that the decision had not been inevitable but had been a calculated one. Had the AEG felt that the priority lay elsewhere then Ward Z would not have been staffed. It had been a difficult choice for the AEG and the priorities memorandum had prompted the Group to have a rethink. The CANO sympathised with the CADO and conceded that in many respects he was right: Ward Z was a hospital service development and represented another blow for dentists and community health services. The CANO maintained that when so little money was available, decision-making and priority-setting became arbitrary, a view which contrasts sharply with that expressed by many officers, and by the memorandum, that a period of economic stringency provided a unique opportunity for rational reappraisal. In the CADO's opinion, priorities were decided on the basis of 'custom and habit', and the hospital service was receiving funds per usual. This seemed to him to indicate that there was, as yet, no real integration in the NHS.

At the PRC meeting at the beginning of June, it was

agreed that the balance of development monies for Year 2 should be made available to open the remainder of Ward Z. The report before the committee recorded the CADO's dissatisfaction with the way in which dental services had been neglected but this had no effect on the final decision, or at least on the formal ratification of a decision already effectively taken by the AEG.

Although no additional funds were forthcoming, both districts in Beta were asked by the AEG to submit revised priorities in respect of their requests for DF in order that the AEG would have an up-to-date appreciation of the situation. Both DEGs were aware that their lists of requests would end up as little more than paper exercises since DF did not exist to fund them. But in the words of one DA

> 'it behoves us as managers to have priority lists of developments if suddenly there is an influx of money; it may be given to us in a hurry and if we're not prepared for papers to be distributed for discussion and priorities to be determined, then I would suggest we're not managing. We've got to up-date all the time'.

Despite gloomy predictions, some funds did materialise, but for nonrecurring purposes only. Most of the money came unexpectedly from slippage in the capital building programme which resulted in a short-fall around December, thus enabling the board to re-allocate £70,000 from the programme to other purposes. But it was a case of choosing schemes which did not attract running-costs and most of these were self-selecting. The other proviso was that schemes had to be completed by the end of the financial year. The Secretary said it was essential to spend all available funds since it was 'not good to persuade staff to economise and then be £100,000 underspent'.

The position in Alpha over DF in Year 2 was similar to that in Beta except that there were no DF to allocate. However, it was agreed that submissions would be sought from the two districts in order to allow extended consideration as to the distribution of any funds that might materialise. The present position allowed no room for manoeuvre since the board was committed to additional expenditure which came close to the anticipated DF for Year 2 (as a result of national policy decisions and the requirement to fund the running costs of completed capital schemes).

As requested, the districts drew up their lists for submission to the AEG. District B adopted a new approach to staffing developments. Instead of the usual practice, whereby the DEG asked for requirements from heads of departments and so on which were then itemised on lengthy lists, usually with a minimum of supporting data, to be sifted through, it was decided that the newly appointed District Personnel Officer (DPO) and District Management Accountant (DMA) should jointly produce the basic information for each development proposal before the lists were considered by the DEG. In this way, the DPO and DMA were interposed between those delivering services and the DEG, and acted as filters for development requests.

The adoption of this new procedure was, in large part, the result of the DPO's disapproval of the existing arrangements. Furthermore, with the separation of finance and administration, it was necessary to try and match the needs of finance to the needs of the Service. According to the DPO, 'we never had to do this before because at BoM level it (i.e. finance and administration) was a joint post' (i.e. Secretary and Treasurer).

The DPO and DMA prepared forms designed to elicit all useful information about a particular request for additional staff, including a fairly exact statement of priority. Heads of departments were asked to state how a particular request stood in relation to other developments for their departments or functions, and were also asked to indicate the repercussions on the service if a development was not implemented. Data were also requested concerning the reasons for a request (e.g. increase in workload, development of service, change in work methods, or change in regulations/statutory requirements), the cost implications and details of what duties the post entailed. In addition, heads of departments were asked to indicate any savings that might accrue from the implementation of a development. The aim of this development-processing exercise was to feed the DEG fuller, more complete, information because, in the past, supporting data had tended to be too subjective. The DPO and DMA, by their own admission, were attempting to inject some rationality into the allocation of DF by examining the lists 'with a fine tooth-comb' before they were submitted to the DEG. The two officers had no executive authority, their task being to advise the DEG. If there was an argument between finance and services then this could only be resolved by the DEG.

After receiving the lists from the DPO and DMA, the DEG's task was to decide which items were to be referred to the AEG. As in Year 1, most of the developments were directed towards filling gaps in services (i.e. 'adding to existing stock'), and only one or two, like the request for ward housekeepers, represented a development of the service. When asked which of the district's priorities was the most important and what would happen if DF were received, the DA replied he did not know - he simply could not say. The DEG would have to review all the A+ priorities and then decide. It would be far from straightforward, especially since this first meeting had been unreal because no DF were likely. Therefore, the DEG was not in a corner. Only when it was cornered did the fighting begin; otherwise there was no need to take harsh decisions.

In Alpha, no staffing developments were undertaken in Year 2 beyond those already agreed to which had been carried forward from Year 1. There might have been some scope for allocating DF had not a second nursing crisis arisen (the first, it will be remembered, occurred in Year 1), this time in district A. It was reported to the PRC that there had been a substantial increase in hospital nursing staff numbers in the district over the two years since reorganisation. Out of an overall increase of 245 nurses (from 1,286 to 1,531), 160 were attributable to developments authorised by the board, or to national agreements arising from, for example, the Halsbury report on nurses' pay. Of the remaining 85, 60 were funded but were not in post in April 1974, leaving an unfunded balance of 25 nurses, i.e. 25 in excess of the figure for which funds were available. The Treasurer stated that, because of his position, his advice could only be to restrict the number of nurses by 25 since any increase over the establishment figure would result in a pre-emption of the small amount of DF anticipated for Year 3. The pre-emption would amount to £70,000 if the nursing establishment were allowed to grow, and this would, of necessity, mean that other developments, including the commissioning of certain capital schemes, could not be implemented.

The CANO, not surprisingly, dissented from this view and supported the establishment figure of 1,531, arguing that it was still below the pre-reorganisation establishment figure of 1,573, which would entail a further 42 nurses. Moreover, he had understood that funds were available to finance this figure (i.e. 1,531), although this now appeared not to be the case. In the view of all the nursing officers, the original higher establishment figure was needed to provide a reasonable standard of nursing care, although the figure still fell short of the establishment which would emerge from an application of the Aberdeen formula.

The PRC agreed that the necessary funds should be made available to finance a hospital nursing staff establishment of 1,531 (which included the 25 in excess of available funds), and the committee noted that this decision would result in DF for Year 3 being pre-empted to the extent of £70,000 which would mean that other developments which had already received board approval could not be implemented.

This incident caused a split in the AEG, with three members against keeping the establishment level at the figure of 1,531, and one in favour. Because a consensus was not possible, the PRC, as mentioned, had to decide between the two choices put forward by the CANO on the one hand, and the remaining three members of the AEG on the other. The Treasurer was particularly concerned at the way in which the decision had been taken in complete isolation, instead of being taken after a review of alternative developments which the board might prefer to fund, or even after a comparison with nursing ratios in other areas. In his opinion, had the decision in favour of nursing been reached after an examination of all possible developments on which resources could have been spent, then that would have been more rational (akin to the process outlined in a rational model of decision-making described in Chapter 3). But this had not happened and the decision, the Treasurer felt, had been taken on irrational grounds and for emotional reasons. The PRC's decision was unanimous in part, the Treasurer thought, because nursing aroused passions - there was a widespread feeling that nurses were important and that the NHS depended on them for its very survival. They were regarded as the backbone of the Service.

The episode undoubtedly placed strains, themselves the outcome of a stagnant economic situation, on the consensus management concept. The Treasurer claimed that whereas in a normal growth year the CAMO, for example, could have agreed to an increase in nursing staff and still have had access to funds for services under his management, now that nursing had received DF at the expense of all other services, the CAMO was under fire for 'selling out' to nurses.

This concludes the description of the allocation of DF over a two-year period in Alpha and Beta. It is now time to stand back from the fray in an endeavour to make some sense of events in the two health boards.

CHAPTER 6

The Allocation Process: An Assessment

In presenting an analysis of the allocation process described in the last two chapters, this chapter begins with a discussion of the importance of DF, and proceeds to examine the constraints operating on decision-makers. As revealed in the descriptive chapters, decision-makers in Alpha and Beta operated inescapably within numerous constraints which largely shaped the decision-making environment. Later in the chapter, the coping strategies, or 'aids to calculation' (to borrow Wildavsky's term) (1), adopted by decision-makers to enable them to make sense of their environment in a situation of uncertainty are isolated.

IMPORTANCE OF DF

The real importance of DF lies in the fact that they are the only guaranteed source of 'new' (i.e. committed) money that a health board receives. The only alternative source of free funds is to effect savings in the remainder of the budget which is already committed to existing services. A DA in Alpha maintained that DF were important because:

> 'many people regard them as the answer. But if we're doing our job we should be looking at services to divert funds that are not being used properly at present, that is, redeploying resources within the Service. I don't think we've spent enough time on

this in the past. The cry has always been 'we need more' instead of standing back and asking if we're using what we've got properly'.

In fact, as was illustrated in Chapter 5, it is extremely difficult to rationalise services in this way, however desirable it may be. The Secretary of Alpha argued that redistributing resources meant:

> 'stopping a service of some sort or other, or reducing a service. It can be done, but it's not easy; the room to switch existing monies isn't very great. The main medium for changing direction is through DF, or through some large project, say, a capital scheme with revenue consequences, which brings revenue money with it'.

DF are even more important at a time when community health services are regarded as a priority for development. The Secretary explained:

> 'People accept that if you do have to change direction it is more towards community care and this, by its very nature, does not bring with it so many large-scale projects. Health centres are the only development in this category, but they don't offer the same chance of switching from hospital based to community based services. So DF are the main way of doing it. It's a small percentage but it can make a difference ... The effect has to be cumulative rather than emerge in any one year. It is the only way you can move, unless you can shut down services and use the money for something else'.

In contrast to community health services, most developments in clinical services come through building schemes. 'There are individual appointments but a lot come through opening new hospitals'. In other words, when DF are stretched or in short supply, it is community health services which inevitably suffer most. Hospital services can continue to expand, albeit at a slower rate, through centrally funded schemes.

Although both Alpha and Beta, and the boards that responded to the questionnaire, were all agreed on the significance of DF, the importance of, and reliance placed upon, them can, to some extent, be linked to the size of a board and to its catchment area for patients for particular services. For example, the CANO in Beta claimed that DF were especially vital

> 'in a small area such as ours where, financially, we have very little room to manoeuvre because of the size of our budget. We have been able to recruit staff so there's no 'slack' in the nursing budget and yet our ratios are low, particularly in hospitals X and Y ... which historically have taken patients from all over (this part) of Scotland and are much bigger than we (in this area) require. We've still got to staff them and any move towards improving psychiatric or MD services in this area depends totally on our development money. We can't start community services because we've got no money to engage community nurses. We can't take them from existing staff because the ratios are so low - dangerously low in the MD unit. So development monies are certainly vital to nursing'.

Like other officers, the CANO agreed that there were other solutions to the problem of providing a better service than reliance on development money. But, certaintly until the onset of 'low growth', DF were easier to come by than better bed occupancy, more efficient use of staff time and so on. Administrators, as they themselves freely admitted, relied upon continuing growth as a means of postponing awkward decisions which would have involved full use of their management skills, like, for instance, monitoring the effective, and efficient, utilisation of existing resources, both financial and manpower, and taking corrective action as required.

Responses to the questionnaire corresponded closely with data obtained from Alpha and Beta. All ten boards found DF to be indispensable, several of them identifying limitless demands on the Service as being a primary reason. One board noted that 'the demands of the public for extensions and improvements of health care and the abilities of the health profession to provide it are limitless'. Not surprisingly, in view of Alpha and Beta's experience, several boards commented on how difficult it was to provide funds for developments by making savings on existing resources.

A final observation is that the importance of DF was directly related to general views about planning that exist in the NHS. Towell (2), for example, claims that planning 'is still tending to be seen as mainly concerned with ordering priorities for the use of any extra resources made available' (emphasis added) rather than a means of redeploying existing resources or altering priorities within these.

'MORE OF THE SAME' OR NEW DIRECTIONS?

While no one disputes the importance of DF for the provision, by health boards, of services where the margin for manoeuvre is narrow, there is a problem when it comes to deciding how the funds should be used. Essentially, two options confront decision-makers: either DF can be used to plug gaps in existing services (i.e. improvements and/or expansions), or they can be used to shift the direction in which a board is moving (e.g. a switch from institutional to community care). It is normally obligatory to choose between these options, being rarely possible to attempt both simultaneously. Moreover, in the long term, implementation of one strategy prohibits taking, or makes it extremely difficult to take, action on the other. This dilemma faced consensus management teams at area and district levels constantly, but never more so than during the period of activity over the allocation of DF.

Officers were well aware of the conflicting demands which, in some way, had to be reconciled. The necessary choices were made more difficult because of the limited DF available. The CAMO in Alpha commented on this dilemma:

> 'When there are so many deficiencies, you tend to have to patch and really do what seems to be the most urgent in whatever field there is pressure, rather than consciously neglect to do something. DF are spread pretty thinly and anything terribly major can't be done'.

Despite this short-term approach to DF, decision-makers tried not to lose sight of mid- and long-term developments they would like to see come to fruition. Yet, focusing on the short-term could act to preclude the realisation of longer term aims. The pressures operating on decision-makers were such that they were forced into a reactive, as opposed to an anticipatory, posture. A DNO in Beta maintained that the allocation of DF in practice amounted to 'reacting to events', and a DA in the same board argued that there was 'no rational, objective basis for allocating DF and determining top priorities out of several mutually competing ones. A great deal depends on the persuasiveness of the case put forward'. A DFO in Alpha echoed these comments. 'In the past, before the DEG, I always felt that the person who shouted loudest got it (i.e. a share of DF). It wasn't always based on pure need or priority but because that person waved the shroud better than somebody else'.

In deciding allocations on the basis of either improvements/expansions, and/or providing a new service, many considerations have to be taken into account. Sometimes the sequence of events complicated matters. For example, as the Secretary of Alpha pointed out, requests for staff might start off as developments but end up as absolute necessities.

> 'The problem is that by the time one considers these requests, the additional member of staff that has been requested to cope with the existing workload is not a development as such because the workload has increased so much that we're entitled to have a consultant (or whatever) almost as of right. A large number of requests reflect existing increases in workload. They are not new developments, but are a response to workloads over which there is sometimes no control. One is caught up in the momentum of the thing. It's all very well to say that the situation should never have been allowed to reach this stage, or that the board's hands are tied and that it was forced into a corner. If patients come forward they have to be treated. This is why I want to build up the community side. It's less expensive and is the best economic bet. It's the only way to throttle off the demand before it reaches the hospital. Thereafter, most of the

additional medical posts can usually be justified in terms of existing workloads. This is the way it works: two consultants begin; after one year, they wonder why things are so hectic, look up the figures, see they're treating so many more patients, and put in a request for a third consultant. At this stage there's not too much you can do about it'.

The dilemma is that by using DF to increase current staff establishments (i.e. 'more of the same'), resources are being committed which could have been put to other, perhaps more effective, uses (3). If the trend is to reinforce existing patterns of care through additional appointments, then altering the status quo becomes progressively more difficult. The dilemma does not pass unacknowledged. As the Secretary in Alpha put it, 'what does one say to a consultant? Does one say, "as soon as you're doing more work than you ought to be doing, stop?" What does one mean by stop? If patients present themselves they've got to be seen'. The CAMO in Alpha, while admitting that this problem existed, added: 'sometimes it's resolved for you in that you just can't continue to expand the existing service because of lack of facilities. It's not simply a matter of getting more staff'.

At best, allocations of DF reflected a compromise between, on the one hand, simply plugging gaps in existing services and, on the other hand, initiating new services where possible. Incompatible elements within these two allocation strategies gave rise to tension. Often there was no choice open to decision-makers and a compromise was not possible. Pressures arising from existing services presented officers with little, or no, alternative but to plough more funds into them to relieve the pressures. The CANO in Beta stressed that allocations of DF were a response to requests which amounted to:

'a 'shopping-list' of deficiencies and pressure points. We don't have a long-term goal or direction in which we're going. Pressures are on at this very moment. I don't think that's right, I think it's inevitable. There has been a tendency to say, 'well we're waiting for the programme planning groups and the Scottish Health Service Planning Council to come up with the answers'. That worries me a bit for a variety of reasons. They may come up with the answers we don't want or haven't had. Far more important is the fact that they are not going to come up with anything very quickly. We really should be planning over the next decade in broad, general terms. But then the pressure to do that isn't there because all our development monies are needed for first-aid or are committed to various projects already in existence'.

An additional problem, revealed in Chapters 4 and 5, was that DF might be allocated to a mix of improvements and new developments but that, at the last minute, plans were thwarted by the flare-up of a crisis, such as occurred in both Alpha and Beta over nursing staff establishments. Attention to crises of this type required switching DF from proposed developments. A DA in Alpha expressed the dilemma facing administrators vis-a-vis short-term pressures on the one hand, and long-term strategy on the other, in the following terms:

'You've got to look at the immediate need. For example, if I'm overweight I go to the doctor; he says in the long-term I should lose weight but I also need my appendix out. Obviously the immediate thing that requires attention is the latter but the long-term view must be kept in mind. Where possible, resources must go towards achieving the long-term goal. But if a crisis arises or the service is in danger of deteriorating, then resources must be diverted to that'.

Most of the allocations over the two-year period studied amounted to a response to pressure points arising from existing services. Officers were quite certain about the need to attend to immediate pressures but far less clear about what long-term strategy they should be following, if any, or, indeed, how far this should override short-term considerations.

SPREAD THINLY OR ALLOCATE IN A LUMP?

A further tension point in the allocation of DF had its origins in the strategy chosen to allocate them. There were two strategies, both of which cut across the improvements/expansions, or new services, dichotomy: (1) the strategy of spreading DF thinly in order to give something to everyone (<u>fair shares</u>); and (2) the opposite strategy of channelling the bulk of DF to a particular development (<u>priority-setting</u>). The priority-setting strategy could refer either to allocation decisions taken to bolster the <u>status quo</u>, or to decisions to start new services (which usually required a substantial injection of funds). Often, however, when lump sums were allocated to developments in existing services, these decisions were not so much the outcome of priority-setting as such (i.e. in the sense of officers reaching a deliberate decision when faced with a genuine choice), but more usually the outcome of a quick response to sudden crises where officers could see no alternative but to bring these under immediate control. The fair shares strategy, on the other hand, was confined to expansion/improvements to existing services ('more of the same').

Both Alpha and Beta tended to pursue the fair shares strategy, even if they did so rather reluctantly. The Secretary (Beta) explained:

> 'In the past, everyone has tended to parcel out amounts to the A priorities. The aim has been to meet all the As, with the result that everyone has got something and was reasonably happy. I've always been well aware that the role of the AEG to the board was to say 'we've failed in this channelling out of development money as a percentage to every department each year. The practice should cease'. The only way to improve the Service is to channel the whole of our monies into a particular area which is so obviously underfinanced that the only way to sustain it is by doing this. There should be less and less of little bits of money spent on a clerkess here, two nurses there, and an engineer somewhere'.

But the Secretary appreciated only too well the obstacles lying in the path of such a switch in strategy. The problem remained

> 'What do you do when faced with requests for development monies largely for additional staff which came in this smallish board to just under £1 million last year? There are so many understaffed areas and so many which should be strengthened. Is there something to be said for just trying to improve a little bit here and there?'

The adoption of a fair shares strategy was also a response to uncertainty. As a DA in Beta commented, 'the difficulty is deciding what is a priority over and above all others'. Evidence available to judge the relative priority of claims for resources was limited and most services could advance claims for special consideration for one reason or another. It is not so much the setting of objectives for the NHS which is problematic but the determination of priorities, that is, deciding which objectives should receive proportionately increased resources.

The DA in district Y (Beta) said that allocating DF was an arbitrary procedure, adding that 'putting all the funds into one sector might be of little use since it might still be wide of the mark and ineffective'. This is not to imply that the DA was making out a case for saying that it was more rational to employ a fair shares strategy but, as he proceeded to argue, 'this would seem to be more effective in that people are prepared to accept a little bit of the cake. But I don't think it's good management. This is where I'm in a bit of a dilemma'.

Although several officers in Alpha and Beta expressed their preferred allocation strategy of concentrating available DF in a particular area, the decision to act in this way was sometimes forced upon them, rather than arrived at through choice after discussionsof the options (that is to say, it was <u>not</u> an example of priority setting as such, since decision-makers were faced with no practical alternative, but an instance of non-decision-making) (4). Over-spending on the nursing budget in both boards over the two years required the bulk of DF for two of the districts to be channelled into nursing, despite the fact that the original intention had been to allocate available monies according to a fair shares strategy.

How DF are allocated, and to what purposes, depends to some extent on the planning capabilities of health boards. The specialist expertise in Alpha and Beta lay in the field of physical planning; service planning was the responsibility of the two AEGs (programme planning groups were also involved in planning but on a longer term basis), but administrators at this level are not trained planners and lack the necessary skills. Their experience and expertise derive from the day-to-day administration of the NHS, even at area level where a more strategic outlook is supposed to prevail.

Planning necessitates choices which reflect a commitment, however flexible the approach adopted, to certain broad aims. In the view of the CANO (Beta), planning means

> 'that we have to decide that geriatric care, or care of the mentally ill, or whatever has priority for that particular year, and it gets the bulk, or all, of the available resources and everybody else does not get very much. At present, I don't think we are indulging in long-term planning in the AEG. Although we tend to say that it's (i.e. the allocation process) based on real priorities, I think certainly once it gets into the broad category of nursing the tendency at the present time is for each little corner of nursing to get a bit. They get a bit mainly because they need a bit but I think we're simply bolstering up a service which is unsatisfactory - we're bolstering it up by another couple of nurses or something but we're not really tackling a particular area of care and providing the resources which will allow, for example, geriatrics to be looked after as well as they might be at home. We tend to fool ourselves at the moment if we think we really are financing priorities. They are priorities in the sense of low staffing ratios and so forth, but inevitably each bit of nursing gets a bit of money at the present time. We're not tackling any major programme'.

Part of the problem identified by the CANO occurred because allocations of DF were approached in input oriented terms rather than in terms of output. 'We're not saying, for example, we'll institute a sensible programme of care for the mentally ill which would involve a nursing component'. Rather, resource allocation was looked at 'in terms of different heads of expenditure, additional staff numbers, and so on'. A Secretary of one Scottish health board wrote (5)

> 'the reorganisation of the service clearly presents an opportunity of adopting a more systematic approach to planning. There is little doubt that, in the past, planning has been largely piecemeal in character and aimed primarily at increasing the supply of staff, buildings etc.'

The last two chapters have provided sufficient evidence to show that the planning of services by Alpha and Beta tended to be confined to dealing with the annual financial increment to service spending - DF. The great bulk of running costs of services continued much the same from one year to the next. It was only the increment that could be used in the short term to alter the character or distribution of services, both by correcting imbalances between services and by satisfying pressing demands from staff. A similar conclusion was reached by Brown _et al_ (6) in their study of Humberside AHA in England. Planning was felt to be useful if the cash was there to meet the requirements (what the authors call the 'development syndrome'), but was of little use if no additional cash was available. In the latter case it was seen as an 'academic exercise'. By planning in this context is meant not a rational procedure akin to that outlined in Chapter 3, but a political dialogue between decision actors involved in allocating resources.

Numerous constraints, both political and structural, inhibited and hindered the introduction of different approaches to resource allocation decisions. These approaches may be seen as part of the attempt, which began in earnest with reorganisation and was, as has been noted, a fundamental theme of the 1974 reforms, to attain the synoptic ideal.

CONSTRAINTS (1) EXTERNAL

Two main sets of external constraints operated to restrict decision-makers' freedom of manoeuvre. They were observed at: (a) the interface between health boards and local authorities responsible for personal social services; and (b) the interface between health boards and the SHHD.

(a) Health Board/Local Authority Interface

Although integration has occurred between primary care, hospital care and community care, personal social services remain under local authority control (7). There is much overlap between the two sets of services and, inevitably, policies pursued by one set of agencies can have an impact on the other. While it has not been the purpose of the present research specifically to observe liaison arrangements between health boards and local authorities, aspects of this relationship, or lack of one, crept into the decision-making process over DF. According to official policy, if a health board wishes to ease pressures on the hospital service, one way to achieve this is to expand community care services. Moreover, re-organisation of the NHS was, in part, intended to facilitate such a shift in health care priorities. Comments from administrators cited in preceding chapters indicate that they too saw the future development of the NHS as lying in this direction. Yet, there were few visible signs of close co-operation between health and local authorities in Alpha and Beta. Decisions taken independently by one authority could have repercussions on policies being pursued by the other. For example, home helps are an important element in any policy shift from institution-based to community-based care, but they come under local authority control. Cuts in local government expenditure (which took effect in Year 2) had an adverse impact on the provision of home helps which made it considerably more difficult for health boards to speed up discharges from hospitals, particularly among geriatric patients requiring nothing more than a little support.

It was reported in Chapter 5 how most of Beta's DF

in Year 2 had been allocated to the opening of an orthopaedic surgical unit, despite the conclusions of a review of orthopaedic surgery carried out by a working party of the board that the pressure on existing beds was caused primarily by geriatric patients who remained in hospital owing to a lack of alternative facilities either in the hospital sector or in the community. It was argued that if this problem could be solved then the number of beds available for medical cases would probably be adequate. The chief obstacle to solving the problem was the inability of the board and the local authority to agree on a policy for the elderly. In the report's words, 'the involvement of local authorities in the care of the elderly must influence the provisions which the health service requires to make'. More home helps and the provision of day centres would relieve the need to provide inpatient accommodation.

Patients suffering from mental distress were also in need of improved community care. In the case of Beta, there were two large hospitals for the mentally ill and mentally handicapped. As was shown in the two previous chapters, their staffing needs, particularly in nursing, were voracious. Once again, action in this area depended largely on policies pursued by the local authority. The report noted that the bed complement of the two hospitals was over and above the needs of the area but that the main factor which would ultimately affect the requirement for beds was the scale of the provision of facilities in the community, among which were local authority day centres. A similar situation prevailed over the provision of facilities for the mentally handicapped. 'In this field, as in the psychiatric field, the question of the involvement of the local authority makes it difficult to assess exactly what provisions the health service should make on its own'. Since the hospital for mentally handicapped patients was 'grossly overcrowded', the aim, according to the report, should be to reduce the number of patients accommodated. This required local authority action to which the only alternative, perhaps as an interim measure until longer term changes began to take effect, was to increase substantially staff/patient ratios to improve immediately the level of care. This was the course followed in the allocation of DF. Had close co-operation existed between Alpha and Beta and their respective local authorities, it is reasonable to assume that this might have been reflected in different uses being found for at least a portion of DF at the disposal of both boards. While it is not possible to be certain, it is unlikely that there would have been the same pressures to boost staffing levels if other means were being pursued which would have alleviated the causes of these pressures. However, faced with these pressures, and with no other options readily available, decision-makers had little choice but to accede to some of the demands for more staff.

Although the above examples have been drawn from Beta, Alpha experienced similar difficulties. Regardless of particular health boards, the key to shifting the burden of caring for long-stay patients from relatively expensive hospital care to the community has always been the social services. Yet it would appear that local authorities are no closer to the NHS than before reorganisation. The current attempt to roll-back public spending may be expected to drive them still further apart. If this happens, Scotland could suffer more than England where joint planning between health and local authorities is encouraged through joint financing. The arrangements allow the two sets of authorities to contribute jointly, in agreed proportions, to the capital and revenue costs of schemes, the cost of which would normally fall wholly upon local government. The health authorities' revenue contribution extends only over a limited period of years, at the end of which the local authority has to carry the full running costs. So far in Scotland there are no plans to introduce joint financing although pressure is mounting for an initiative similar to that operating in England and Wales (8). This difference between Scotland and England (and Wales) is illustrative of the general difference in approach to health planning between the two countries, with greater central intervention a feature of the English arrangements.

(b) Health Board/SHHD Interface

Despite considerable freedom to allocate resources, health boards are, at the same time, subject to certain national policy decisions which it is their duty to observe and implement. The two examples encountered in Year 2 were family planning and junior doctors' pay. In times of growth, this pre-emption of funds by national decisions was disguised through additional monies coming from the SHHD; but during periods of low-growth, as in Year 2, and as a consequence of cash limits, boards were expected to find the revenue for national policies from within their own allocations. This outcome, therefore, tended to confirm the view of many officers that during periods of resource scarcity the SHHD intervened more readily in the affairs of health boards although this intervention did not mark fundamental change of policy by the Department. Most officials within the SHHD agreed that the tight resource situation had led to greater Departmental involvement in health board affairs which, in turn, had acted to curtail boards' autonomy. Prior to the economic difficulties, the SHHD funded additional major capital developments by allocating sums of money over-and-above the basic allocation of DF. Because major schemes brought money with them for running costs they were, as Alpha's Secretary said, an 'easy way of developing the service (and) of financing additional staff'. According to Beta's Treasurer:

> 'if you find your place in the major programme you then get the identifiable additional running costs guaranteed. This would release DF for the community services, if you were lucky enough to have major schemes for the hospital service within the centrally-financed programme. If you were not involved in this programme then DF might be needed to finance the running costs of schemes within the board's own ordinary capital programme'.

Consequently, schemes in the major programme have their running costs protected while other schemes, including many in the community services, have to find their way through the ordinary programme and share in the competition for DF. Moreover, at a time of resource constraint, those capital schemes which either effect savings or have minimal running costs will be favoured over those which generate additional running costs even if, from a board's point of view, a scheme coming into this last category has top priority. This could result in a channelling of capital funds towards certain types of activity only, especially after the SHHD had warned boards that if the running costs of new buildings were greater than those of the buildings they replaced, improvements in other sectors of the Service would have to be foregone.

Therefore, the climate in which administrators within health boards operated was affected by Departmental action, even if this action exerted an indirect influence on the decisions boards took, rather than a direct one. For instance, as noted in Chapter 5, in Year 2 boards were requested by the SHHD to give priority to schemes with no running-cost implications. But this rather contradicted the Department's attempt to shift the balance of health care provision towards the deprived sectors and towards community care. It was in such a contradictory, stop-go environment that administrators had to make decisions which, individually, seemed innocuous enough but which, cumulatively, had a considerable impact on the development of services. The Secretary of Beta maintained that all the board could do was react to events.

> 'Forward planning is very difficult. We need clear-cut advice. (It's) a stop-go situation at present and planning is almost impossible. Our capital programme is cut, then we're told money is available to help ease the unemployment situation. But we have to choose projects with no running-cost implications, which means we are giving priority to schemes which don't really warrant it. How can you plan on this basis?'

However, the relationship between the SHHD and health boards is not akin to a superior-subordinate one. It is in many ways more complex, a consequence primarily of its ambivalence. Popular mythology suggests that administrators in health boards are incapable of exercising any autonomy they may possess for fear of upsetting the Department. This is too simplistic a view of the relationship. As the Secretary of Alpha explained

> 'the Department has always been very reluctant to instruct a hospital or health board - this is not their way of doing things. It's always guidance. The Department doesn't want to give instructions or be drawn into a situation where it would have to do so. The Department allows us a lot of autonomy'.

Apart from issuing advice and guidance, the SHHD imposes certain limits on boards through the laying down of conditions of service, salaries and staffing norms. All of these are decided upon in conjunction with the appropriate professional bodies who are largely responsible for negotiating national agreements with their inevitable centralising tendencies (9). Health boards are free to operate within these limits. In certain spheres, and for certain lengths of time, the SHHD maintains a firm grip on the policies pursued by boards. For instance, after a public outcry following reorganisation about 'excessive' bureaucracy in the NHS, the SHHD (following the DHSS in London) declared a halt on recruitment of administrative and clerical staff. For certain new posts, boards had to seek SHHD approval before making appointments if these exceeded the figures applicable on a particular date (10).

On the evidence obtained from Alpha and Beta, and from general observation, while it would be incorrect to conclude that a high degree of centralisation exists which totally excludes local variation and priority-setting, there are indications of a shift in the relationship between the SHHD and health boards, with greater interest by the centre in health priorities becoming a feature of it. This has emerged with reorganisation and as a response to resource constraints and related political pressures. In many ways, the relationship combines a mixture of centralising and decentralising tendencies, which accounts for the paradoxical situation whereby health board officers and civil servants make contradictory statements which are, in a sense, both correct. For example, while many officers at board level, and civil servants in the SHHD, denied that the centre's influence was increasing, it was accepted by some that the existence of fifteen boards did facilitate intervention by the Department; a counter-argument reached the opposite conclusion, namely, that it was much more difficult for the Department to throw its weight around when there were fifteen authorities to confront. To complicate matters further, and to compound the ambivalence, officers may resent inroads into their allocations of DF because of national policy decisions, while, at the same time, welcoming an increase in central influence over priorities both as a means of giving boards a lead and a clear direction, and as support for them when they were faced with strong opposition from the professions over, say, hospital closures.

It must be emphasised, however, that pervasive central involvement in health board affairs should not be equated with central <u>control</u> over what boards do. In any relationship there has to be give-and-take and when it comes to DF, for example, boards are not obliged to allocate them in particular ways. This is not to suggest that boards are wholly free in their decision-making activities in regard to these funds; there are many internal constraints operating which, if anything, can be more restricting than central intervention. Health board autonomy from central control is not meant to imply autonomy from other influences operating internally at board level.

CONSTRAINTS (2) INTERNAL

The environment within which officers in Alpha and Beta operated imposed numerous constraints on their freedom of action. Eight, in particular, played a crucial role in determining the allocations of DF.

(a) <u>Existing Services</u>

Alpha and Beta, like all health boards, were stuck with services inherited from the past. Allocations of DF were not concerned, solely, or even primarily, with services starting from scratch - there is never a 'clean slate'. Once services were established, a board was committed to maintaining them, particularly when they rapidly gathered momentum and were regarded as indispensable. Mention has been made of the two large hospitals in Beta for those suffering from mental disorders. The staffing demands, particularly for nurses, of these institutions seemed insatiable and placed a severe strain on Beta's DF. Faced with such pressures (and Alpha had its share), officers could choose between immediate, though temporary, relief, or longer-term solutions. The preference was to provide immediate relief to ease pressure points which meant forever tinkering with staffing ratios, adding to them in small increments as funds and staff became available. Alpha's Secretary pointed out that attempts were also made to begin to shift the emphasis of health care away from the hospital service although it was far from simple in practice because as demands built up on, for example, consultants it was not possible to stop patients from being seen. The episode over the orthopaedic surgical unit in Beta in Year 2 is a good example of this tension at work and illustrates the seductive pull of existing services. Inevitably, existing services wielded a powerful, if not a decisive, influence over allocations of DF. In a setting where 'priorities by decibels' represented almost the only viable allocation strategy pursued by both boards, it was from existing services where the loudest voices and the noises inevitably came. New departures could not compete in such an environment.

(b) Time Lag

By this constraint is meant developments being funded in the present which had been inherited from the past, usually from former health authorities before reorganisation. In short, DF, in some cases, were already committed before they were even allocated. There was, for instance, the new maternity unit in Beta which received funding although it went against the priority recommendations in The Way Ahead. It was, in the jargon, 'an ongoing commitment'. Yet, in the new economic climate, when maternity generally was being cut back to release resources for other purposes, perhaps the maternity unit ought to have undergone a change of use to cope with some priority area such as the elderly. But, according to district officers, the unit could not be altered because the board was too deeply committed to it. In this way, time lag hindered the redeployment of resources and narrowed down the options open to decision-makers.

Other examples of time lag concerned the nurse staffing crises in Alpha and Beta. These had their origins in the days before reorganisation when BoMs gave nursing officers a free hand to acquire staff. Not surprisingly, such permissive acts led to overspending on the nursing budgets which prevented other developments from going ahead as financial order was restored.

(c) Real Time

This was an obvious constraint which affects decision-makers in any organisation. Nevertheless, it remained a crucial one since a fairly rigid timetable was adhered to in allocating DF. Generally, the quicker decisions were taken, the sooner funds could be disposed of, staff appointed and the less chance there was of funds remaining unspent at the close of the financial year and then being hurriedly spent on items of dubious priority. But a tight timetable reduced the time available to administrators, particularly at district level, to prepare detailed cases supporting submissions for DF with the result that many allocation decisions were taken on the basis of crude information and subjective criteria of assessment. It was mentioned in Chapter 4 how both DAs in Alpha had complained in their memos accompanying the development lists that they had had insufficient time to consider the requests as thoroughly as they would have wished and that they had not been able to put them in exactly the priority order that they would have liked. The real time constraint permeated the remaining constraints described below.

(d) Information

This acted as a constraint in two ways: either there was (1) a surfeit of information which was just not being made use of (for reasons of information overload, or poor dissemination), or (2) a shortage of particular kinds of information. In other words, the constraint comprised a political component and a technical component. By political is meant the ability of individuals, or groups, either to withhold potentially useful information, or their reluctance to make use of data in a way that might threaten particular interests. Technically, information was sometimes available but was ignored, or not gathered, because of the time and/or cost required to put it into an appropriate form. The political problems involved in gaining access to available data and in persuading professionals to act on them, and the technical problems involved in assembling data inevitably resulted in greater weight being attached to the persuasiveness of a particular officer in putting a case for a development. A further problem, which is elaborated below under priority-setting, was that there were limits to the usefulness of information in assisting decision-makers when deficiencies of equal need had been identified among several sectors. Masses of statistics are routinely collected in the NHS but they do not assist in making the fundamental decision of whether to establish, or expand, one service as against another.

In deciding allocations, the main types of data used were: staff/patient ratios, staffing numbers (reference was frequently made to a document published annually, Scottish Hospital Costs (SHC), for comparisons with other boards; if a particular board was unable to attain the ideal staffing norm, as invariably was the case since staffing norms were usually considered to be unrealistic in terms of practical attainment, then SHC acted as a guide as to how a particular board was faring by allowing comparisons to be made with comparable hospitals, etc. in other boards), workloads, waiting-lists, and bed occupancy rates. These types of data tend to be rather crude and do not necessarily provide reliable indicators of need, possibly reflecting other factors like, for example, inefficient staff output. Staffing norms, in particular, are widely believed to be unrealistic and virtually unattainable within existing growth rates, yet they provide various professional groups with powerful bargaining weapons. Klein (11) has argued that the derivation of establishment figures is often obscure and is the result of pressures and counter-pressures rather than of rational planning. It is, in any case, extremely difficult to arrive at objective staffing norms since there are, in practice, wide variations between hospitals, even those in the same category.

(e) Consultation

Consultation is a particular feature of the reorganised NHS and it is a lengthy and complex process. In allocations of DF, the AEGs in Alpha and Beta were obliged to consult widely before reaching final decisions on DF. Seeking the approval of professional advisory committees was time-consuming even if it was a good investment. The Secretary of the SHHD observed at a conference in late November 1977 on the reorganised Scottish Health Service: 'I think we have paid an inescapable price in slower decision-making and many man hours spent in discussions with perhaps a disappointing outcome in terms of the value of so much earnest deliberation'.

(f) Consensus Decision-Making

Like consultation, consensus management is a key feature of the reorganised structure. Reaching unanimous agreement could take time. More significant, perhaps, it also presented difficulties for particular officers who were unsure of their precise role. For example, a DA in Beta found himself in a dilemma over the allocation of DF in his DEG. He was confronted by three professional officers, the DMO, DNO and DDO, all of whom claimed that their particular developments were top priority. What the DA wanted to know was who the arbitrator was? It could not be him because he had to reach a consensus with two of the professional officers, the DMO and DNO, and his coordinating role did not extend to an ability to arbitrate between various requests. Moreover, he was himself a professional officer with direct responsibility for ancillary staff. In the previous structure, lay boards performed this adjudication function, with the Secretary and Treasurer (a joint post) putting the choice to the BoM for decision. But in the absence of a lay board at district level, if proposals cannot be agreed upon by the DEG then they must be referred to the area and, failing agreement at that level, to the board as a last resort. Districts were naturally reluctant to refer to the area matters that lay within their jurisdiction since an action of this kind could be interpreted as incompetence on the part of the district team. The ever-present risk of having to refer decisions to the AEG worked to ensure that DEGs, wherever possible, reached their own decisions within a consensus framework. This did not solve the dilemma outlined by the DA, and it could be argued that developments were approved that might have received closer scrutiny had there been an individual, or a board of lay members, who could have performed this adjudicatory function. The AEG was ill-equipped to undertake this task for reasons outlined in Chapter 4 (e.g. too remote; lack of time, knowledge etc.), and the health board itself had to cope with so much business that it was unable to even give a great deal of attention to a scrutiny of development lists which had already passed through district and area teams. It is just possible, then, that the consensus framework tended to reinforce the strategy of fair shares in the allocation of DF, although many other factors were also involved, including the inheritance of allocation practices and routines from the previous structure. There was no direct evidence to substantiate, or refute, the proposition, only that of a circumstantial kind.

(g) <u>Organisational Fragmentation</u>

The fragmented nature of health board decision-making and administration precludes the comprehensive approach required for the effective resolution of problems affecting priorities and the allocation of DF. Within the policy triad - health board, officers, advisory groups - there were numerous divisions, and each component of the triad had its own particular interests. Recent fashions in health service organisation have centred on increased functionalism and specialisation among the providers of services (12). The management structure exemplifies the fragmentation present. In Alpha and Beta there were three management levels - area, district and sector - and within each there were numerous competing interests. The spread of functional management has created further fragmentation and has increased the difficulties in reaching consensus decisions. The complexity of the management structure is, to some extent, a consequence of its fragmented nature. The area/district relationship, and the tensions arising from it, has received some attention. Perhaps these tensions were most evident in the role conflict arising from the AEG/DEG interface. District officers performed a dual role with many inherent incompatibilities. For example, in a particular situation, should they remain loyal to the DEG of which they were members, or to their area counterparts to whom they were directly accountable? As was shown in the account of development fund allocations, there were occasions when district officers had to choose between these conflicting demands. The very existence of such tensions did nothing to improve area/district relations, particularly in the case of districts eager to overcome their essentially subservient position in the hierarchy. The consequent suspicion, and competitive posturing, induced by this fragmentation led to decisions on DF which were perhaps not always in the interests of health care for the area as a whole, although they may have been in the interests of particular district officers and functional managers anxious to gain what they could for their district or function. The approach to savings is a clear example of how organisational fragmentation could act as a constraint from the area's viewpoint.

(h) Priority-Setting

The allocation of DF was about choices and priorities - inevitably so when funds were not available to do everything that was desired. Officers in Alpha and Beta, especially at district level, experienced great difficulty in placing requests in order of priority, which probably explains why most of them were placed in the A category, with few in the B category and fewer still in the C category. While there were problems in deciding between these categories, that is, which developments should be A-rated, B-rated or whatever, the knottiest problems arose when attempts were made to decide within categories, particularly the A category since most developments fell into this. The choices were of the order of whether a dental officer should come before a nurse, or whether a domestic should come before a doctor. Officers faced a dilemma over which categories of staff were more important at a particular point in time and, as one DMO said, 'one could never be absolutely certain that one had one's priorities right' - 'guesstimates' played a large part in the process. A DFO in Beta commented that in making decisions of this kind there was no formula; it had to be done through personal appraisal of each case. He found it an almost impossible task, especially when it was not possible to identify benefits that were clearly linked to particular developments.

'How do you begin to evaluate the value of the services of, say, one more community nurse as opposed to improved nursing services to the mentally handicapped? To look at a set of accounts is just a record of where the money was spent. When you apply a cost-benefit approach, you can locate the cost but what's the benefit? You don't know. The best you can do is to say that the yield from that expenditure was so many inpatient days, so many operations in that specialty, so many visits by a health visitor, etc. Are you any further forward? How do you determine standards, or what output to expect? If, for example, one community nurse in her average day does eight visits, and another community nurse does fifteen visits - what does it mean? It's the quality of the service that is important but how do you measure this?'

Decisions about priorities between different disease, or dependency, groups posed complex problems since they required cross comparisons to be made between different groups of the population who were suffering from different conditions, and they raised fundamental value questions, such as, for example, how do decision-makers compare providing care for an elderly person with undertaking cardiac surgery for a middle-aged man suffering from heart disease? Decision-makers in Alpha and Beta faced this kind of dilemma, albeit indirectly, since there concern when allocating DF was with additional inputs, that is, more staff, rather than with particular client-groups or service categories. In such circumstances, it was all too easy to reduce priority-setting to a matter of life-and-death criteria, i.e. to 'waving the shroud' (13). As a District Management Accountant from Beta explained, the difficulty in the NHS was that many decision-making and resource-allocation problems were political, by which he meant that there were rivalries among groups within the NHS each of which was intent on pursuing its own particular interests. He was referring also to the inability to apply a rational model of decision-making, as outlined in Chapter 3, to an environment which was so divided and fragmented with competing interests and loyalties. It was a clear case of the demands of rational analysis being simply too great despite efforts to achieve it.

COPING STRATEGIES

In the absence of hard, objective criteria, or of any overall strategy, for allocating DF, decision-makers had to make some sense of their environment and make some attempt to structure it in order to render it manageable. They achieved this by devising, and operating, their own strategies for allocating DF. These did not eliminate all conflict but they enabled decision-makers to reach decisions quite quickly within a framework which provided them with the necessary justification for reaching a particular decision.

Wildavsky (14) has written that in resource-allocation decision-making, aside from other complexities, there

> 'remains the imposing problem of making comparisons among different programmes that have different values for different people. It involves deciding such questions as how much intensive care units are worth as compared to geriatric facilities, health education, staff, etc. No common denominator among these functions has been developed. Officials discover they can't find any objective method of judging priorities among requests ... (It is)

necessary to develop mechanisms for helping men make decisions that are in some sense meaningful in a complicated world'.

These are among the problems with which health board officers in Alpha and Beta grappled. As has been suggested (15), 'If it is sometimes easy to know what should not be done, it is seldom clear what should be done, or what can be done'. Decision-makers faced with situations of complexity and uncertainty 'rely on decision rules, rules of thumb or standard operating procedures' that make decision-making manageable (16). In Alpha and Beta four decision rules, or coping strategies, were deployed by decision-makers at different times and in varying degrees. The strategies are considered separately for analytical purposes, although in practice there was much overlap between them.

(i) Who Has Done All Right So Far?

If some group had done particularly well out of DF in a previous year, it would probably receive less in a subsequent year on the grounds that it was now someone else's turn. Examples of this strategy were quite common in Alpha and Beta. The laboratory service in Alpha was allocated fewer DF in Year 1 on the grounds that it could not continue to expand at the same rate as it had enjoyed in past years. To some extent, the emphasis in both boards on community care in Year 1 was a consequence of the application of this strategy. The CANO in Alpha maintained that although community nursing had been favoured in Year 1, in Year 2 it might be the hospital service's turn. In other words, although the marginal shift towards community care can be seen as an example of innovation (see next section), the shift could very easily be short-lived if, after a time, officers (like the CANO) felt that this sector had received more than its fair share of available monies, in which case the tactic of 'turn-and-turn-about' would be employed, a variant of the fair shares strategy.

(ii) Who Has Had Too Much in Relation to the Rest?

During development fund allocation meetings, particularly in Year 1, a great deal of horse-trading took place. If some group appeared to have received an 'over-generous' allocation at an early stage in the negotiations, some of this might be creamed off at a later stage in order to ease pressures elsewhere. For example, in one case funds were initially allocated for three physiotherapists; by the end of the meeting this had been reduced to two. These often random, seemingly arbitrary, and usually last-minute, decisions were sweetened with the recurring comment: 'well, at least it's an improvement in the service'. In this way officers 'satisficed'. They did not try for the best of all possible worlds, but tried to avoid the worst in order to get by.

(iii) Who Has Over/Underspent?

If a particular head of expenditure was overspent, then it was unlikely to receive additional funds (with the possible exception of nursing for reasons already given) as a sanction against further overspending. If underspending occurred, questions were likely to be asked concerning the appropriateness of further allocations if the possibility existed that they would not be spent during the financial year.

(iv) Who Will it Hurt Least?

When deciding upon allocations of DF, officers might be anxious to try to narrow down the number of competing claims by eliminating those staff categories which might be able to do without an injection of funds. For example, in Alpha, district A's original development lists for Year 1 featured a request for eight domestic staff at a mental hospital. The request did not reappear until after a visit to the hospital by a team from SHAS. In anticipation of the team's report, the AEG asked the district to review its decision not to fund this particular development although the DEG had decided previously that it was not a priority and could afford to wait.

These four decision rules, or coping strategies, all

formed part of an over-arching allocation strategy, fair shares. As mentioned in an earlier section, DF were invariably allocated on the basis of fair shares all round, rather than on the basis of directing all available funds to one particular development. There were of course a few exceptions to this general rule, such as the opening of a new orthopaedic surgical unit in Beta in Year 2. Furthermore, crises could alter development plans and involve the bulk of available monies being channelled into an activity to 'put out the fire'.

The fair shares strategy had the effect (whether intended or unintended makes little difference) of perpetuating the existing pattern of service provision which, correspondingly, lessened the chances of introducing any major innovations in the direction taken by particular services. And even if shifts in service delivery patterns and priorities did occur, as in community care, these tended to be the result not so much of some rational, objective assessment of need (however defined), but the outcome of more subjective criteria like political fashion, public pressure, resource scarcity, and so on. Just as many of these pressures frequently worked to produce decisions which reflected a commitment to existing services, so, too, could they result in decisions of a somewhat different nature (17).

A fifth strategy, bending the rules, was of a different order from the rest since it was not so much concerned with setting priorities (not directly at any rate) as with assisting district officers to circumvent the idiosyncracies and rigidities of the budgeting system, and to enable them to pursue the interests of their particular districts as vigorously as possible. Various tactics were available. For instance, according to a DA in Alpha,

> 'If you're underspent in a certain category, you're quite free to divert that temporarily. You can't swing it away forever - that is more a policy matter. We should be able to make temporary changes - to play it by ear, or off the cuff, as the year's progressing'.

Another tactic concerned wage awards.

'When a wage award comes along we claim that automatically. I think everybody takes a little bit of licence when they are making these bids. If you don't overdo it you'll get away with it. You claim a little bit more than it will cost you in practice. This is yet another way of gradually building up and getting yourself into a better financial position, which then allows you a bit more freedom. It's a very small thing but if you're doing it with the nursing award and when the clerical and administrative award comes along and you're making a bit every time, it all helps. You can't ask for the moon. They (i.e. SHHD) can't pin you exactly and if you don't go over the score you can get away with it. This applies when you're bidding for new capital schemes. You've got to make a bid for the running costs. If you do a little over-estimating, it's OK. Any administrator is trying to get as much money as he can. The controls that are placed on us lead us to adopting such strategies'.

These, and other (18), tactics show that officers, particularly those at district level, saw one of their chief tasks as obtaining as large a share as possible of DF from the area for their own purposes.

THE SCOPE FOR INNOVATION

Despite all the problems and constraints facing decision-makers, they are occasionally able to make changes in policy. There are numerous, though often scattered, pressures for policy change and sometimes these, either separately or combined, are powerful enough to bring about breaks in precedent. Changes in public opinion, the appearance of crises, and the availability, or non-availability, of financial resources are all capable of giving an impetus to shifts in policy.

All the allocations of DF may be said to have been incremental, although a few were more incremental than others. In Alpha and Beta there were no dramatic policy shifts, although the example of community care services illustrates that it is unwise to generalise about the total impossibility of bringing about change of any kind in the NHS. Change may be rare for the reasons already stated, but the emphasis on community care, particularly in Year 1, while not resulting in major differences in the quality of, or balance between, services, was an example of how change could occur at the margin, as distinct from the more common practice, or routine, of adding to an existing base. In short, it marked a departure from the ratchet principle governing most allocations, whereby existing services were merely added to each year and the commitment to an ongoing system of service provision was reinforced.

A number of factors accounted for this policy shift in favour of community services. First, many administrators were acutely aware of a feeling among those providing community services that reorganisation was nothing more than a takeover of the entire health service by the hospital service. Health boards were looked upon as old RHBs in disguise. An obvious way of overcoming these fears and suspicions was to channel resources into community services in order to show the good faith of the administrators and to prove to those working in this sector that the administration had their interests very much at heart.

Second, a related factor was that the community services inherited by health boards from local health authorities in 1974 required urgent attention since many had been seriously neglected and were substandard. Boards simply could not ignore these deficiencies which put community services in the category of 'poor relation' to the well-endowed hospital service.

Third, and perhaps most important, the political climate in the mid-1970s was well disposed to a policy initiative of this kind. By 1974, community care had become politically fashionable as well as economically attractive. As the economic situation continued to deteriorate, while the cost of running the NHS continued to escalate, the appeal of community care as a policy priority increased. Economic reasons and motives prevailed although these were laced with humanitarian ideals. It was claimed to be cheaper to treat people at home, instead of putting them into costly institutional surroundings (which remains to be proven, although there is increasing evidence that questions this assertion) (19), and it was also widely maintained that institutionalising patients was demoralising and dehumanising. With national politicians, and a number of pressure groups, favouring community care, albeit for different reasons, officers in Alpha and Beta responded accordingly. They had a clear objective to move towards (outlined, for instance, in the priorities memorandum) and one with which they agreed. Local and national considerations converged on the same objective and officers perceived community care as offering some kind of solution to, or relief from, numerous near-intolerable pressures on the hospital service which would be likely to worsen in view of the limited resources that would be made available to the NHS in future years.

These factors, then, played a significant, if not a decisive, part in creating a climate favourable to community care services. Provided a certain climate exists, that is, one where there is broad consensus among all interested parties, then there is a greater chance of change being possible. Although the emphasis on community care was not dramatic, or sustained, the shift that occurred is worthy of note. Nationally (i.e. Scotland), in 1974/75, hospital services accounted for over 72% of total expenditure with the community health service for over 5%; in 1975/76, the figures were over 70% and over 6% respectively; in 1976/77 the figures were just under 70% of the total and just under 6% respectively; finally, in 1977/78 the figures were just over 70% of the total and under 6% (i.e. 5.62%) respectively (20). The drop in expenditure on the hospital service has been largely due to declines in capital investment. In Alpha and Beta, spending patterns mirrored national trends, although there were slight variations between the two boards. In Alpha, a breakdown of the districts' developments authorised for funding in Year 1 revealed a small swing to community health services. While the emphasis on these services varied between the two districts within Alpha, there was an overall area-wide bias towards the community sector. The position in Alpha is shown in Table 6.1 which comprises a review of spending trends on revenue account over the four-year period since re-organisation, 1974/75 to 1977/78. Although the proportion of total revenue expenditure on community health services increased by a mere 0.3% (a large part of this increase went on the cost of a new Domiciliary Night Nursing Service) between 1974/75 and 1975/76, the table shows that an overall commitment to community care was not sustained beyond Year 1. Between 1975/76 and 1977/78, spending on community health services began to fall until in 1977/78 it was 0.1% below the level it had been in 1974/75 and this at a time when the priorities memorandum stated that continued improvements in community health services were desirable. As Table 6.1 shows, expenditure on the hospital service fell during this period in line with the national picture. The sector which increased its share of available funds throughout the period was primary care. It has been pointed out elsewhere that primary care services are largely demand determined and are not susceptible to administrative control. Moreover, the status of GPs as independent contractors reduces the scope for influencing their numbers. Expenditure on drugs is determined mainly by considerations of demand and professional practice. It is more than likely that a combination of these factors was responsible for increased spending in this sector. The increase in pharmaceutical costs in the period 1974 to 1978 was caused in part by the introduction of new family planning provisions in 1975 which included the prescribing of oral contraceptives by GPs. Because of the contractual relationship, primary care services constitute an open-ended commitment financially; the SHHD makes available funds to the level of the actual expenditure involved.

TABLE 6.1 Percentage Distribution of Revenue Expenditure on Hospital, Community and Primary Care Services 1974/75 - 1977/78 (Alpha)

	Hospital*	Community	Primary Care
Percentage Distribution	%	%	%
Year 1974/75	64.9	8.3	24.6
Year 1975/76	63.7	8.6	25.4
Year 1976/77	63.0	8.5	26.5
Year 1977/78	63.1	8.2	26.5

* Total includes ancillary services, associated services and specialist services costs.

Source: Financial Reviews (Alpha)

A closer look at revenue expenditure in Alpha between 1974/75 and 1975/76 suggests that community health services did rather well in terms of real growth in Year 1 (see Table 6.2). In the hospital service, the real growth rate amounted to 4.1%, while in the community and school health services the growth element amounted to 9.9%. In terms of overall percentage increase in revenue expenditure, community health services did proportionately better than hospital services by 4.1%.

TABLE 6.2 Revenue Expenditure - Percentage Increase 1974/75 - 1975/76 (Alpha)

	1974/75	1975/76	% Increase
Hospital Services	£11,955,377	£15,993,106	33.8
Community & School Health Services	1,512,371	2,086,158	37.9

Source: Financial Review (Alpha)

In Beta, as Table 6.3 shows, the revenue expenditure position was broadly similar to that prevailing in Alpha. However, the situation in regard to community health services was more static; there was practically no movement between this sector and the hospital service with the exception of the year between 1974/75 and 1975/76 when spending on community services fell by 0.1% There were greater fluctuations between the hospital service and primary care services over the four-year period. Nevertheless, Beta was able to achieve some redistribution of resources within the hospital service. Between 1974/75 and 1975/76, total hospital running costs showed that there had been a movement of 1.1% in resources from acute hospitals to long-stay hospitals. This swing was chiefly brought about by nursing staff increases at the two large hospitals in the area. However, while this movement was in line with national policy in regard to long-stay hospitals, it resulted not so much from a consideration of all the alternative options facing officers (i.e. a rationally calculated decision) but from the staffing crisis at the hospitals to which officers had little alternative but to attend. Moreover, this movement was not sustained between 1975/76 and 1976/77 when spending patterns reverted to their 1974/75 position. There was a slight improvement between 1976/77 and 1977/78.

TABLE 6.3 Percentage Distribution of Revenue Expenditure on Hospital, Community and Primary Care Services 1974/75 - 1977/78 (Beta)

	Hospital*	Community	Primary Care
Percentage Distribution	%	%	%
Year 1974/75	67.6	6.2	19.5
Year 1975/76	65.7	6.1	20.3
Year 1976/77	65.2	6.2	21.3
Year 1977/78	65.8	6.2	21.1

* Total includes ancillary services, associated services and specialist services costs.

Source: Financial Reviews (Beta)

Although the case study only covered two out of the four years since reorganisation, a review of spending trends in Alpha and Beta over the four-year period suggests an overall picture of policy maintenance with only occasional slight shifts in expenditure between priority and non-priority services which are not sustained beyond a year or so. In Alpha, the small swing to community care was an example of innovation (at least in relative terms) but it was not sustained beyond Year 1 of the research. It is not easy to account for the fluctuations. Obviously the shortage of DF in Year 2 and beyond was a factor which doubtless added to the difficulties and general organisational inertia which worked against any sustained policy change. On the other hand, the fluctuations (which were also apparent in Beta although not in the community services which presented a fairly static picture) probably reflected the potency and persistence of a fair shares allocation strategy coupled with its turn-and-turn-about variant. Whatever the explanation, clearly policy change at local level was minimal and not enough to disturb an overall national picture of policy stasis. Nonetheless, the micro shifts that did occur were indicative of some discretionary activity at local level.

This analysis goes against that of those who seek a distinction between 'creeping development' and 'consciously chosen development' (21). In practice, there was considerable blurring of the two. Change over time can occur but it is not the inevitable, albeit gradual, consequence of development fund allocations. For the most part, change is a product of the same political system and set of relationships that on the whole operate to prevent change from occurring. To this extent, change is uneven, disjointed, selective rather than sequential, eschewing 'continuity of direction' (22), and is only likely to succeed when it accords with the interests of those groups whose needs and actions tend to dominate the policy agenda at national and local levels within the NHS.

All that can be concluded about the scope for innovation is that a favourable climate at national and local levels can facilitate change, albeit limited and temporary, and that such political factors count for more than attempts at innovation through rational analysis and problem-solving. However, a more potent factor in decisions on the allocation of DF would appear to be the concept of fair shares which renders policy change unlikely, or, at best, temporary as each year brings with it fresh demands from existing services which result in a thin spreading of resources.

CHAPTER 7
Conclusion: Policy Implications for The NHS

The concluding comments are in two parts. First, conclusions are drawn from the case study of the allocation of DF; and second, there is an attempt to draw some overall conclusions from the research in the light of recent developments in the NHS. Since the research was completed, the Royal Commission on the NHS (set up in 1976) has reported (1) and the Government has proposed changes in the structure of the NHS (2). The second part of this chapter considers the implications of the research findings for these proposals.

CONCLUSIONS (1) THE CASE STUDY

As a general observation, it would not be unfair to describe the decision-making process in Alpha and Beta concerning DF as consisting largely of administering and maintaining a system rather than of making fundamental changes in it. Much of the discussion about change, and the need to set new priorities which may have led to large-scale changes, tended to remain at the level of symbolic posturing ('coffee table chat') rather than find itself translated into actual allocation decisions. Of course, significant changes would take many years to achieve and it is possible that a new climate had to emerge before action could proceed. The rhetoric of planning and better resource use was perhaps intended to achieve this. Not that change was impossible within the confines of the existing allocation procedures, but it was rare, often of short duration and a product of the same set of political relationships which most of the time inhibited change. Developments largely meant 'more of the same' through improvements and expansions rather than significant new departures. In general, decision-making was biased overwhelmingly towards attending to the arrangements of the health care system rather than towards making the arrangements, a consequence in part of the numerous constraints operating on decision-makers and a state of affairs aptly captured by the notion of 'non-decision-making'. This mode of operation largely accounted for the way in which the hospital service continued to absorb the bulk of available resources. The basic expenditure patterns had their origin in the days before the NHS was created and they had not been questioned over the years, that is, not until the SHHD'S SHARE report. Even so, SHARE is not concerned with resource-allocation within health boards but only with allocations between them.

The purpose of this research has been to discover why the system operated as it did at local level, and to do this through finding out how decision-makers themselves explained and accounted for their actions. The decision process surrounding DF was complicated - it involved large numbers of people at different levels of the health board structure all representing different interests. The process was also fragmented - not only were there two main tiers involved in the allocation process, areas and districts, but there was an array of other bodies whose requests for developments had to be sought, and whose views on the proposed allocations were required. It was noted in Chapter 3 that the organisational setting in health boards was a plural one, comprised of groups competing against each other (for part of the time, at any rate, covertly if not overtly), and having different views about the nature of health, health services and their place in these, rather than sharing a common view on such matters. In addition to complexity and fragmentation, there was disjointedness - decision-makers did not follow a plan as such but were more inclined to follow their instincts which had been sharpened over many years of experience. Resources were allocated in ways that seemed most feasible at the time, rather than in ways that always reflected what were supposed to be priorities (as laid down, for example, in the SHHD's priorities document); 'putting out fires' absorbed more attention and DF than the initiation, or development, of what were supposed to be board priorities. At best, officers were engaged in a juggling act and, if possible, tried to do a little of both, that is, put out fires <u>and</u> allocate small amounts to new developments (like the domiciliary night nursing service in Alpha).

The problems posed by a decision process that was complex, fragmented and disjointed were not caused by a lack of information <u>per se</u>, since some information did exist to assist those responsible for allocating DF. Whether this information was assembled correctly, or used to its best advantage, were different matters of a political, as well as technical, complexion. Information is a highly valued commodity the possession of which confers power and status. Accordingly, the acquisition, and use, of data in decision-making cease to be purely technical activities and become part of a political process. For example, staffing norms exist in nursing and various paramedical groups are moving in a similar direction. Although norms are regarded as assets in that they provide decision-makers with firm guidelines and clear criteria of staffing need, there is, nevertheless, a problem concerning their reliability, not to mention their practicability, in certain situations. Invariably, the norms tend to veer towards the ideal rather than being geared to solving existing problems in an acceptable way. This was why administrators in Alpha and Beta often made comparisons with staffing levels in comparable boards rather than keep to the established norms with their inbuilt escalatory tendencies. The ability of norms to assist decision-makers was of limited utility when, for example, understaffing was present in several areas of nursing and all these gaps were listed as A priorities - how was one then supposed to decide whose requirements were the most urgent? If a health board had a low level of nursing staff in a mental hospital and a low level of community nursing staff, the problem became one of deciding which had the higher priority. Faced with these dilemmas of choice, administrators coped in various ways, but particularly in their use of coping strategies such as those described in the last chapter. Submissions for DF always outstripped the funds available. Therefore, pruning and trimming became necessary so that the lists of requests for funds could be brought into line with available resources. These were the principal weapons in the armoury of administrators engaged in the allocation exercise. The reference to weapons is not inappropriate - the allocation process, according to one DA, could be quite bloody!

Development lists could best be described as 'shopping-lists' of deficiencies - they were not linked to any specific policy objectives, or to any broad development strategy. Lists were compiled from requests received direct from staff, from heads of departments and through other channels. From the start, therefore, decision-makers were engaged in a reactive process as opposed to an anticipatory one. Moreover, because it involved asking staff about their wants, needs, shortages and pressure points, the whole exercise merely served to raise expectations which administrators then had to try and satisfy. Not surprisingly, perhaps, some members of Alpha's AEG were not altogether happy with the development lists system. Did the lists reflect 'need', or 'demand' and how reliable were they? The AEG was sceptical of the claims contained in the lists. It was not simply that the 'insurance principle' was at work, whereby requirements were deliberately overstated so that some requests might receive funding, but that the opposite might also be occurring, that is, the 'resignation principle', whereby the lists understated requirements because staff had not bothered to submit requests in the belief that they were unlikely to be successful in having any of them met. If, indeed, this was what was happening, then it was an argument in favour of the fair shares allocation strategy because, by attempting to give as many people as possible even a little of what they asked for, then it was more likely that they would not despair of the system and would submit a reasonably fair assessment of their requirements. The extent to which requests reflected need rather than demand, and vice versa, has never been an easy question to answer where health services are concerned. Since it is widely accepted that 'need', a relative concept, is professionally defined (3), the dividing line between need and demand is extremely hazy.

In reviewing the lists of submissions, officers concentrated on each submission in isolation, without relating it to any particular goal or objective. There were some odd exceptions but the overall tendency was to take decisions in a piecemeal fashion. While this approach prevented any examination of the total situation in regard to health policy, and of alternative ways of allocating resources, it was simpler for a decision-maker to 'separate' problems in this way. At the same time, there did exist an inertia whereby it was easier to agree to new appointments rather than to look beyond the immediate need for additional staff in order to examine the form of care provided and possibly alter this. As has been stated several times already, new staff appointment decisions were important because little-by-little they altered, or, more usually, reinforced, the pattern of care and the board was then committed to this pattern with the result that altering the status quo became increasingly difficult. The restriction of vision on the part of officers was a consequence of the numerous constraints which impinged on them and made up the environment within which they operated. Some of these, like pressure of time, were technical; others, like the pressure to be fair and to allocate DF in such a way that as many groups as possible derived some benefit from them, were more political. District B (Alpha) was aware of some of these problems and, in Year 2, adopted a different approach to compiling development lists and ordering priorities. However, because of the absence of growth monies it was not possible to determine how successful the new procedures were. They certainly did not obviate the need for choices between competing claims of equal merit.

Although administrators utilised a number of strategies to structure their complex, fragmented and disjointed environment, a major conflict, which was implicit rather than explicit, remained concerning whether DF should be used primarily to change the direction of services provided, or whether they should be used instead to plug gaps in existing services. If you did one, you had considerably less freedom to do the other; an emphasis on plugging gaps made it increasingly difficult to bring about policy shifts because existing services were being continually reinforced, thereby adding to the annual clamour for more resources which emanated from the vested interests associated with existing services. The dilemma over which allocation strategy to choose may be termed policy stress, since neither was strictly compatible with the other. In practice the dilemma was resolved by using DF to remedy deficiencies since there was constant pressure from existing services for more resources. Pressures to initiate a change of direction were not heard so loudly, or clearly, and usually came from outside the Service. Policy stress could also occur when there existed two concurrent policies which were not strictly compatible with one another. For example, to shift the emphasis towards community care was not compatible with the appointment of more consultants, if these were going to establish more firmly the institutional orientation of the Service.

The general rule governing the allocation of DF was that 'something is better than nothing'. A policy of appeasement was preferred, the aim being to keep as many people happy as possible. Administrators, on the whole, were ambivalent about the merits of this approach. On the one hand, they believed it to be unsatisfactory and that the only way to improve a service dramatically was to channel the whole of available DF into a particular area which was obviously underfinanced; in short, there should be less and less of little bits of money spent here and there. On the other hand, the nature of the environment within which administrators operated was hostile to such an approach but rather well suited to a fair shares strategy which was tailor-made to the requirements of a situation where resources were not available to cope with all demands placed upon them and yet where there were numerous equally competing demands to be placated with the monies that were available. As administrators argued, what do you do when there are so many understaffed areas and so many which require to be strengthened? Consequently, there may well be something to be said for trying to improve a little bit here and there - it was a 'rational' response in the circumstances then prevailing. While in theory other policy options might have been usefully explored, in practice, administrators, even at area level where policy planning was supposed to occur, were predominantly concerned with short-term considerations and the solutions they reached, and the allocation strategies adopted by them in response to particular pressures, reflected this 'crisis management' approach to allocation decisions. A DA summed up the views of many officers when he acknowledged that various inefficient practices, like differing lengths of in-patient stay, existed but that 'the officers had done nothing. There was no need. When 'new' money came in annually, there was no incentive to question existing practices or resource usage'. Even when, in Year 2, DF were reduced, many officers saw themselves performing a holding operation until a period of 'normalcy' returned.

The allocation strategy of fair shares might also be termed the ratchet principle, that is, each group received the same as the previous year only more if possible. Incrementalism is frequently associated with processes of resource-allocation and budgeting which follow this pattern. Schultze (4) argues, in a different context, that most of the individual budget decisions made each year are incremental in nature, and by incremental he means a system whereby budget reviews examine only those items for which increases over the prior year are requested. In the jargon, there are no 'zero-base reviews' - the base for most reviews is the previous year's budget levels. Wildavsky (5) has described a similar process on numerous occasions. For him, and for Schultze too, a non-incremental policy may be defined as one that departs sharply from past practice, or one that requires a large increase (or decrease) in the commitment of resources to a particular service. In resource-allocation processes, the synoptic ideal is impossible to obtain in its pure form, although it is frequently held out as a goal to be approximated as nearly as possible. But, as the account of the development fund allocation process has tried to show, actual budgetary decisions disclosed a somewhat different picture from the ideal. Alpha and Beta, and other boards to judge from their responses to the questionnaire, operated incrementally by restricting attention to small segments of a total problem, comparing a few alternative marginal departures from the existing base and considering only what could be achieved with readily available resources, namely, DF. This strategy is akin to Braybrooke and Lindblom's 'successive limited comparisons' (6).

In his analysis of local government budgeting, Greenwood (7) is concerned with incrementalism as applied to the budgetary process rather than to the amount of change that occurs in the budget, i.e. the outcome of the process. The two criteria he employs to determine whether the budgetary process is incremental or not are the parameters of budgetary review and the mode of budgetary analysis. He found that local authorities operated incrementally since the parameters of review were limited and the mode of analysis was not rational, in the sense of systematic appraisal of consequences and purpose, but political (i.e. non-rational). Greenwood's findings closely resemble those obtained from Alpha and Beta and reported here. Discussion of the allocation of DF was located against a background assumption that there existed (in theory at any rate) a rational model of decision-making in the NHS. Reorganisation of the NHS was concerned, as earlier chapters have shown, with improving decision-making by streamlining the administrative structure and encouraging the application of budgetary techniques which would facilitate the attainment of specific priorities. In particular, financial management skills were deemed important in addition to basic accountancy skills. A rational model presupposes the existence of a consensus within an organisation, or decision unit, among those charged with taking decisions. In other words, so the theory goes, decision-makers share a unitary view of organisational relationships and adhere to a belief that a common goal unites them all. Tensions, or conflicts of interest, if they arise, are dismissed as irrational and are viewed as technical problems. However, in the allocation of DF, rationality in this sense was severely limited by the organisational and political environment which exists at health board level.

Incrementalism which stresses cognitive deficiencies, or technical problems which are intellectually impossible to grasp and resolve, does not suffice as a full explanation of limited rationality. The implication that incrementalism could be avoided, or reduced, if better information was available overlooks the political and organisational dimensions of decision processes. The allocation strategy of fair shares was employed as a means of coming to terms with these dimensions. It was a way of defusing potential clashes of interest by appeasing these interests. The clashes were anticipated by decision-makers in order to avoid, or minimise, them (an example of latent conflict). The commitment to existing services (the ratchet principle), which, above all, governed the flow of DF, was a means of avoiding conflict while recognising, and accepting, the existence of powerful interests. More than this, there was considerable puzzlement and uncertainty about the objectives the NHS ought to be pursuing and how progress might be made towards their achievement. But these reflected political constraints and values as well as information problems. There were, then, obvious political reasons, in the form of vested interests and differing value-systems, to account for DF being allocated in ways that were non-rational if judged by the criteria adopted to denote a rational process of decision-making. In fact, the allocation processes pursued were 'rational' from the viewpoint of those making the decisions, given the constraints within which they worked. Faced with constant pressures arising from existing services for more resources, there were powerful, and convincing, reasons for operating at the margin but no further.

An account of incrementalism which attempts to include political and organisational factors can help to explain why some decisions are more, or less, incremental than others. An example where an attempt was made to alter the <u>status quo</u> in a somewhat less incremental fashion was community care. The focus on community health services in Alpha especially was the outcome of a political dialogue at local and national levels, and not the outcome of rational analysis. Policy-making is to some extent about fashions and fads, like the emphasis on management in the early 1970s throughout the public sector, and while there were particular reasons for the emphasis on community care services, there seems little doubt that the national commitment to this policy option that emerged forcefully in the 1970s had much to do with what Schon (8) has referred to as 'the emergence of ideas in good currency'. He continues: 'underlying every public debate and every formal conflict over policy there is a barely visible process through which issues come to awareness and ideas about them become powerful'. It was pointed out in Chapter 6 that the attempt, which was only temporarily successful, to shift the emphasis in Alpha and Beta from hospital to community care, was an instance of innovation in an environment heavily committed to patching up the status quo. It has been argued (9) that 'the difficulties of identifying and causing change are ... enormous' and that 'it takes particular pertinacity to work for large-scale changes which cannot become quickly visible and hence rewarding to those who have to defer present advantages for the sake of future gains'. Alpha and Beta were not exempt from these pressures.

Significantly, Greenwood (10) argues that, in recent years, local authorities have become less incremental in that they have widened their parameters of review and have attempted to introduce rational analysis into the process. It is likely that corporate management techniques, which have been adopted by local government in a way not followed by health authorities, offer a partial explanation of these developments. Of course, changes might occur in the style of decision-making described in this research project, although at the time of the study it was too early to tell. Certainly the rhetoric among officers was rational, but the reality remained incremental. Admittedly, in Year 2, officers in Alpha and Beta did look at existing commitments and probed their expenditure base to a degree that represented a departure from previous practice. However, from the sporadic efforts in regard to locating savings and reallocating resources it was impossible to conclude whether it was merely a form of tokenism or window-dressing, or whether it marked the start of a fundamental switch in widening the parameters of review and in the mode of analysis adopted in allocating resources. Further exploration of these practices would be useful.

However, what the case study does reveal are the obstacles and entrenched operational routines that will have to be tackled if progress is to be made in equalising service provision within boards. While techniques like management accounting and programme budgeting may better inform decision-making and clarify the choices available, by improving the visibility of allocations, they may also, paradoxically, reinforce policy stasis rather than improve the chances of introducing change (11).

To sum up these reflections on the allocation of DF, it is not being suggested that the process was wrong in some way. Given the constraints operating, the absence of an agreed approach to the problem of deciding priorities and the tremendous problems involved in devising acceptable measures of performance (i.e. outputs) upon which all those providing and receiving services can agree, the processes observed were, in some sense, 'rational'. They were realistic and took account of the <u>political</u> nature of an environment where a number of professional groups were engaged in jostling for a 'slice of the cake'. Any other approach might have been totally unrealistic, impracticable and, therefore, unworkable. Commenting on the operation of the planning system adopted for the NHS in England, a report (12) concluded:

> 'At area and district where strategic planning confronted more immediate realities, rationality seemed less relevant and more tempered by other demands: for example, the upgrading of operating theatres despite a foreseen change of use of the hospital; and keeping an accident and emergency department open despite the continued running of another one nearby, were responses to more immediately felt wants'.

There are, then, multiple perceptions of rationality within settings comprising groups of decision actors at different levels each possessing different responsibilities and loyalties.

POLICY TRIAD

The policy triad comprised the three groups of decision-makers - health board members, officers, professional and lay advisory bodies - involved to some degree in the allocation of DF. Not only were there inter-group tensions within the triad, but there were also intra-group pressures. One of the purposes of the case study was to observe the nature, and extent, of the influence of each of the three elements of the triad on the allocation process.

Clearly, officers were the most active element of the triad involved in allocating DF and they dominated the scene. However, it would be a mistake to equate high visibility and intense activity with an equal measure of influence. As officers' own assessments of the nature of the allocation exercise suggested, they were not so much in control of events as reacting to pressures as and when these surfaced. Officers, in other words, and recalling the distinction made in Chapter 3 between the activities of management on the one hand and administration on the other, acted more like administrators than managers. The allocation process over the two years offered ample testimony to the preoccupation with short-term pressures. In addition, officers were constrained by the sheer weight of existing services and the seemingly unstoppable momentum of inherited commitments.

In Chapter 2, the medical profession's special relationship with the NHS was dealt with at some length. It is worth relating this discussion to what actually happened in Alpha and Beta. While there was some direct evidence of clinical autonomy at work in the two boards through, for example, attempts by officers to persuade doctors to review their clinical practices in an endeavour to use resources more effectively and more sparingly, by far the greatest impact of clinical autonomy on allocation decisions was covert and indirect, thus conforming to Lukes' (13) conceptualisation of power. Power, according to this view, does not show up in cases of actual conflict since it is aimed at <u>preventing</u> such conflict from arising in the first place. As long as the interests of those who set the policy agenda (in this case the allocation of DF) are not threatened then a state of latent conflict may be said to exist. Thus allocations of DF did not always reflect directly the wishes and wants of doctors; nor did they arise from some conspiracy on the part of the medical profession to win for itself the biggest share of available resources so depriving other groups in need of them. The process was altogether more subtle. The plain fact is that, in their present established position as leaders of the health care team and as the primary decision-makers, doctors' decisions to treat patients commit resources such as nurses, technicians, equipment and materials. It is individual consultants who, consciously or unconsciously, affect the level and pace of work in the hospital through their 'gate-keeper' function. Of course, once other groups like nurses, and an array of support staff are established, they acquire a momentum of their own and impose additional pressures on administrators charged with allocating resources. But it is the needs of doctors, as initially defined by them, which trigger off the expansion of these other staff categories. Time and again in Alpha and Beta, the appointment of a consultant had a 'knock on' effect on other services. The medical profession may be said, then, to set the agenda of development fund allocations if only by preventing, or hindering, by their very existence and by the terms of their contract with the NHS, the emergence of an alternative policy agenda. While a state directed health system might succeed in nibbling at the edges of these arrangements (see next section), they have remained largely intact to data.

It was suggested in Chapter 1 that it was over-simplistic to subscribe unerringly to the view that politics is about conflict and power. Although power was at work in the allocation of DF, as mentioned above, it did not involve conflict primarily because the very way in which the NHS is organised and operates, namely, as a set of arrangements conceived to provide a range of services to meet a range of 'needs' or demands, inevitably includes certain interests while excluding others. For example, a perspective emphasising health promotion inevitably merits a lower priority in a Service organised around a medical, or disease-centred, model of health based on the interests of the medical profession and other occupational groups. Officers in charge of allocating DF may profess to be exercising power but the narrow range of choices open to them in deciding upon allocations reflects their recognition of what might happen if they attempted seriously to enact dramatic policy shifts. An application of Lukes' concept of power reveals the sheer weight of the acute hospital services which continue to absorb the bulk of available resources so preventing any lasting attempt to shift resources to other sectors. Once services, like those comprising the acute sector, are established, organisational inertia sets in and the pressures to attend continually to them become overwhelming.

Politics, as noted in earlier chapters, is also about puzzlement and uncertainty - 'men collectively wondering what to do' (14). According to Heclo, 'the possession and relationships of power have not necessarily decided the substance of policy' (15). Because decision-makers in Alpha and Beta were uncertain about the likely outcomes of policy shifts, it was much easier to play safe and maintain services along familiar lines. Despite the rhetorical stress on preventive health, and on the alleged desirability of community services, which may have been a substitute for action, there was much ignorance as to what precisely was involved in terms of service impact on client-groups. One administrator (16), for instance, has argued that evidence is lacking which would enable the efficacy of currently fashionable policy moves to be tested. The emphasis on primary care services, he suggests, 'is based more on an act of faith that (these) will be better and cheaper, than on hard evidence that they will be effective in ... reducing or alleviating ... morbidity'. There is an 'abysmal lack of answers' to the question of what is 'effective in therapy and prevention'. There are, in any case, no easy answers. Improved primary care services may ease the pressures on hospitals but then again they may lead to increased referrals. If one attempts to tackle the problem at the other end, by improving the efficiency of resource use within hospitals, there is a danger of 'heating up the system'. Speedier throughput per bed, for example, can lead to more GP referrals which, in turn, lead to increases in the workloads of hospital staff and higher operating costs. Moreover, progress in the spheres of prevention and community care require active co-operation on a sustained basis between health and local authorities and, as has been pointed out, there was not much evidence of this in Alpha and Beta. All these factors served to reinforce a commitment to the status quo.

Compounding these structural pressures is the ability of doctors to apply emotional pressure to win resources. Again, this need not occur in a crude, overt manner because when it comes to matters of life and death, it needs very little pressure to persuade most people of the 'benefits' to be derived from putting resources into life-saving ventures (17). While seasoned officers may hold private reservations about these allocation, they know that the weight of public opinion and media reaction would be likely quickly to reverse a decision that attempted to pursue a different course at the expense, say, of opening a new ward to reduce waiting-lists and ease pressures on existing staff and services. It was considerations like these that, in part, governed Beta's decision to proceed with staffing an orthopaedic surgical unit in Year 2 despite the recommendations of the priorities memorandum which favoured the adoption of policies aimed at the community and the chronic sick. Another factor was that the unit was an inherited commitment.

The influence of officers on development fund allocations while not pronounced was, on the surface, greater than that of the professional advisory structure. But, in view of the arguments above, there is no particular reason why advisory committees should have been influential given that none of the allocation decisions showed significant departures from existing service provision to which professional groups were largely wedded. While there may have been odd grumbles from some quarters about not getting what they considered to be a fair share of available resources for staff, there was no radical policy shift envisaged which would have been likely to antagonise professional bodies and spur them into action. Overall, allocation decisions conformed to traditional professional views about services, the ways in which these should be delivered, and the staffing levels required to deliver them to the desired standard. The influence of lay advisory bodies on the allocation process was practically non-existent during the observation period primarily because LHCs were in the process of being set up. However, from the available evidence concerning the potential of these bodies, their impact on DF was likely to resemble that of board members (18).

The impact of board members on the allocation of DF was minimal. This was consistent with most members' accounts of themselves and their role, and their general feelings of remoteness and impotence (19). The only time board members genuinely found themselves in a position to exert influence on the decision process was when there were divisions within the AEG which prevented a consensus from being reached. But this was a rare occurrence and it only happened once, in Alpha in Year 2, over nursing establishment levels when the matter in dispute had to be referred to the board for decision. In the main, both AEGs presented united fronts to their respective boards which made it considerably more difficult for board members to exercise much influence.

The allocation process, as preceding chapters have suggested, was characterised by a small number of key actors who determined how the funds were to be spent. This group was composed of officers at area and district levels whose task it was to assemble the list of proposed allocations that went forward to the board, via its principal standing committee, for approval. Although board members were presented with opportunities to query proposals, in practice it was difficult to perform such a role when expertise and motivation were lacking (20). Moreover, the allocation process was structured in such a way that it insulated the key decision-makers from lay involvement. The organisational processes surrounding allocations of DF were evidence of this. All meetings over DF prior to the board's pro forma acceptance of the final package were private. In addition, requests for DF were not generated within the board; they, were, in most cases, demands created by staff, what Danziger (21) has termed 'withinputs'. These 'bright ideas' were transmitted up through sector, district to area. Therefore, the operation of the resource allocation process had the effect of insulating those with decision-making discretion, in particular the officers, from public demands, as expressed through board members, and from visibility. Such insulation might just be defensible if the decision process was extremely complex and technical. But much of the process observed involved political judgements concerning what constituted priorities and so on. Subjective criteria frequently governed what was deemed relevant or irrelevant in the way of developments. Significantly, while accepting the value-laden nature of priority-setting, one administrator (22) is of the opinion that the obstacles to meaningful lay participation are so great that 'decisions about priorities will, of necessity, be made by professionals - administrative, medical or political - even if this introduces an element of paternalism'. While these comments are directed primarily at LHCs, whose task it is broadly to represent the views of the public to health authorities by facilitating community action in regard to health matters, they have a direct bearing on the feelings of frustration and impotence experienced by many board members in Alpha and Beta. Given the nature of decision-making over DF, as it has been described, it is perhaps not surprising that many members felt remote from what was actually happening within their own board.

CONCLUSIONS (2) GENERAL COMMENT

Gouldner (23) has written:

> 'It is not the sociologist's task to <u>recommend</u> alternative policies and to insist that some administrative options are 'better' than others. But if he is not a proper catalyst of social change, neither ought a sociologist to serve as a justifier of received patterns, legitimating them with <u>post factum</u> omniscience as the product of 'inevitability'. If the sociologist may not expatiate upon what

'ought to be', he is still privileged to deal with another realm, 'the realm of what can be'.

In this final section, the report of the Royal Commission on the NHS (24) and the Government's consultative papers (there are three papers, one each for England and Wales, Scotland, and Northern Ireland) (25) on proposed changes in the structure and management of the Health Service are considered in the light of the findings to emerge from the case study on development fund allocations.

Since the completion of the fieldwork for this research, the environment inhabited by the NHS has become more turbulent. The state of the economy, inflation, public spending controls and cash limits, private practice and pay beds, the impact of re-organisation, industrial relations, and professions' pay are all factors which have had a corrosive effect on the fabric of the Health Service in recent years. The Royal Commission on the NHS was set up by the Labour government in 1976 in the midst of this turbulence and it reported in July 1979, only by this time a Conservative administration had replaced Labour in office. The new Secretary of State for Social Services, Patrick Jenkin, had firm views on reforming the NHS; as Opposition spokesman on social services, he had expressed on numerous occasions his intention to simplify the structure. Not surprisingly, his ideas became the cornerstone of the Government's response to the Royal Commission's report and, in December 1979, a consultative paper (with counterparts in Scotland and Northern Ireland) was issued setting out the Government's intentions. Final proposals will emerge after the four-month consultation period but legislation is presently going through Parliament (26) which confers on the Secretary of State the power to establish new district health authorities in England. Changes in the Scottish structure do not require legislation. The most profound structural changes will occur in England in view of its complicated four-tier structure; in Scotland it is expected that some amalgamation of districts below areas will occur. Whatever decisions are finally taken, the Government is anxious to proceed so that reforms might be completed by the end of 1983.

With further organisational change in the offing, the insights provided by the case study could be of value in determining the possible impact of reform, even of the limited variety being canvassed for Scotland. But a note of caution must be sounded. The ability to generalise with any certainty from one case study of one particular decision process, which has been observed in two health boards (out of fifteen), is extremely limited. Nevertheless, while the case study is probably unable, by itself, fully to support all the arguments which follow, sufficient evidence emerged from it to substantiate, to some degree, the points made below about the limitations of structural change. Before exploring the policy implications of the case study, it will be helpful to summarise briefly the relevant parts of the Royal Commission's analysis and the consultative papers for England and Scotland since these documents will underpin future changes in the NHS.

THE ROYAL COMMISSION

The Commission's report is a sober and sensible, if at times over-cautious, assessment of the state of the NHS. While accepting that there are serious problems and deficiencies concerning resources and service priorities, it concludes that there is no need to 'feel ashamed of our health service and that there are many aspects of it of which we can be justly proud' (27). Although one of the report's five parts is devoted to management and finance, the Commission believes that these matters 'are essentially secondary to those subjects which bear directly on patient care' (28). It dismisses the desirability of radical change in the structure of the NHS, such as the creation of a health commission to manage the Service at arm's-length from the DHSS, or the transfer of the Service to local government (with the proviso that the question should be reconsidered if regional government became a possibility in England). The Commission favours a 'middle way', namely, devolving responsibility to health authorities and restoring status and authority to hospital administrators. These reforms are believed to be essential for 'good, clear administration' (29). In particular, it is argued that there should be more flexibility in the administrative arrangements (the Commission overlooks the possible incompatibility between flexibility on the one hand, and clear administration on the other), and that the structure needs slimming with only one management level being necessary below region in England (which would continue to exercise responsibility for strategic planning), and elsewhere in the UK below health department (i.e. in Scotland, the SHHD). However, the Commission is under no illusions that its proposals on structure would produce miraculous results. The report states (30):

> 'Abolition of a tier seemed to have assumed symbolic importance and was seen as the universal solution to the problems of managing the NHS. We do not ourselves regard abolition of a management tier as a panacea. There are many reasons for the present difficulties in the NHS and structure is only one of them'.

In its discussion of accountability and the role of health authority members, the report is disappointing and scarcely considers the subject. Yet, as the case study showed, board members experience considerable role uncertainty and have difficulty in holding officers to account. More important than the arguments over selection versus election is the problem of whether board members are able to perform satisfactorily the role prescribed for them and whether, in fact, this role is one for which members are best suited (31). The Royal Commission completely overlooks these questions.

In considering financial management at health authority level, the Commission draws heavily on the work of a team (32) produced at the Commission's request. One of the team's conclusions is that financial control systems are satisfactory in terms of fiscal regularity but that they are 'little used for planning and decision-making in any positive sense of resource reallocation or conscious testing of alternatives' (33). The research team place great stress on more accurate and comprehensive data on patients in order to inform decisions about resource allocation and deployment. They also recommend research to provide 'better measures of need and output' so that 'decisions about resources would be more soundly based' (34). These proposals are commendable but it is important, as the case study presented here has shown, not to overlook the political features which permeate decision-making processes and underlie judgements about priorities and so on. One area where progress might usefully be made is in clinical budgeting since, as the case study again reveals, many resources are committed through the decisions of consultants and their staff although they do not have the responsibility for managing these resources within budgets. The Commission's report recommends experiments with clinical budgeting since 'the clinical decisions that doctors make heavily influence NHS expenditure' (35). In the report's words, 'there can be no such thing as absolute clinical freedom' (36). Of course, doctors are already subject to broad constraints in regard to (a) the total amount of resources made available to the NHS; (b) allocation policies which seek to redress geographical inequalities (e.g. RAWP, SHARE); and (c) allocation policies which seek to direct resources towards particular care groups (e.g. priorities memorandum). Therefore, while 'implicit rationing' (37) of resources by the medical profession still occurs (the case study provides some evidence of this), the existence of 'explicit rationing' (38) cannot be ignored. Indeed, over coming years when DF will probably remain in short supply, the influence of a state directed rationing system (which already exists to some extent in the shape of a national health service) in priorities may be expected to grow as attention is focused increasingly on the use made of existing resources.

THE GOVERNMENT'S INTENTIONS

This section examines the consultative papers for Scotland and England. The Scottish one is obviously of direct relevance in the context of the case study of Alpha and Beta, but the English one is also important since the philosophy underlying the Government's proposals is spelt out at greater length than in the Scottish paper.

The Government sets great store by getting the structure and management of the NHS 'right'. The English paper states: 'If these are not right, then nothing else will work properly' (39). Such a positive emphasis on structural change marks a shift from the Royal Commission's view that too much was generally expected from structural change and that it should not be seen as a panacea for failings within the Service. Central to the Government's plans is a commitment to greater local responsibility to enable services to be more flexible, and more responsive to local needs. However, the consultative paper does not specify how this shift in central-local relations to the local level is to be achieved, beyond proposing between 150 and 200 District Health Authorities to replace the existing 90 AHAs in England. Indeed, given the continued existence of a centrally funded Service which is accountable to Parliament through the Secretary of State, tensions between centre and periphery seem inevitable. Furthermore, the proposals contain some fundamental ambiguities and inconsistencies which threaten to undermine the alleged intention of reform (40). For instance, the stress on flexibility and sensitivity to local needs does not sit well alongside proposals for a strengthened regional tier or for the composition of management teams (41). A more fundamental objection is that most of the proposals refer to hospital services, while community services, primary care services, preventive services and, indeed, the entire 'health field' (42), receive scant attention. Links with other agencies, in particular local authorities, are also played down while great emphasis is placed upon returning authority to the hospital administrator. As if to justify its bias, the English paper claims that integration between hospital and community services 'has been substantially achieved' (43). Available evidence (44), including the case study findings, suggests that this is not so and that if the 1974 reorganisation achieved little else, it alerted people to the fact that health care is about much more than just hospital services.

For all its ambiguity and general vagueness, the consultative paper may assist in moving the NHS in the direction of greater local diversity where flexibility of response is of the essence. This can only be desirable in a policy area where knowledge is imperfect and where 'models of good practice' cannot be imposed from above. As the case study shows, field health authorities already possess a fairly substantial degree of discretion although this occurs in an environment where the centre is, in theory, supposed to exercise control. The fact that it cannot do so effectively adds confusion to, and blurs responsibilities in, an already uncertain and fragmented setting. Also, it may be that health authorities choose not to exercise what discretion they possess because of local constraints of one kind or another. But such 'masterly inactivity' is a problem which the Government's proposals will do little to resolve. Action here rests almost entirely with local health authorities.

While sharing a similar philosophy in regard to the need for simplifying the structure and management of the NHS, in Scotland 'no further substantial reorganisation' is envisaged (45). Area health boards are to remain but 'should work on the basis that the normal structure should be a single district area' (46). In boards like Alpha and Beta the proposal to abolish districts is likely to receive considerable support given that the two-tier structure in these boards led, on occasion, to problems over deciding who was responsible for what.

The two consultative papers, especially the English one in view of the scale of the operation in England, proffer yet further structural solutions to the problems of the NHS. At best they may be seen as not 'more of the same' but 'less of the same' given that they are an attempt to simplify administration and facilitate the development of a Service that is responsive to changing local needs. However, the findings to emerge from the case study suggest that more than structural tinkering is required if real change is to manifest itself, since proposals of the kind put forward by the Government fail to take into account the politics of organisational life. The search for the 'right' <u>structure</u> ('one best way'), as distinct from the right <u>approach</u>, is misconceived. It is an illusory goal, especially if it is thought that once the new structure is in place conflicts and tensions within the NHS will melt away.

A considerable part of the analysis of decision-making and budgeting presented in this book has been taken up with drawing attention to the gap which exists between rational policy pronouncements and the reality which exists in executing these. Reorganisation of the NHS in 1974, based on a rational model of health service management and decision-making, is a classic example of this misconceived approach to social change. Through an attachment to the rational model, the fiction is maintained that decision-making is rational and that it occurs in accordance with a set of clear, objective, technical precepts. The reality, of course, is quite different and far less simple. Moreover, not only does structural change of the kind associated with massive reorganisations serve to disguise the real processes which operate, and to inhibit discussion of the methods actually used to allocate resources, it may even be counterproductive and make the attainment of desired goals more remote. This is because reorganisation itself involves costs (47). Hood (48) has observed that

> 'in the extreme case, reorganisation and ineffectiveness can become causally related: ineffectiveness causes demands for reorganisation, but reorganisational costs reduce effectiveness in the short term, which leads to demands for yet more reorganisation, and so on'.

Such a 'reorganisation complex' (49), or what has been referred to as the 'British Reorganisation Game' (50) has become a feature of the NHS and Hood's observation is particularly apt in the light of the Government's proposals for further structural change. The dilemma is that actions intended to improve administrative performance may fail to do so and, in fact, change nothing of substance, in which case, reorganisation becomes little more than a form of 'tokenism', i.e. it becomes a symbolic response to change which is 'a symptom of the inability to achieve 'deep change'. This type of reorganisation is an attack on symptoms rather than causes' (51). Mant (52) likens the activity to 'a purification ritual', a 'clearing out of dead wood'. The Government concedes in the English consultative paper that 'changes in the structure alone will not be sufficient' and that changes in management arrangements will also be necessary (53). But it is not clear what precisely is meant by changes in management arrangements, apart from a strengthening of management at hospital level, and most of the specific proposals and detail of the paper refer to structure.

Evidence suggests that organisations seem to be harder to change at the bottom than at the top (54), and in practice the field administrative structure may change less than a reorganisation might suggest. But if, as some believe it is, the reorganisation complex is 'a substitute for making choices' (55), in this case in health policy, then it is not surprising that the emphasis should be on structure at the expense of process. While the Royal Commission's analysis recognises the limitations of structural change in the NHS, there is a danger that the Government may repeat some of the errors incurred in 1974, despite the rhetoric in the consultative paper about the need for flexibility and gradualism. As the case study suggests, other features of organisational life in the NHS, not susceptible to structural solutions, may be more important in securing a shift in priorities.

Of course structure is important but its impact on behaviour and outcomes is overstated. Structural change can achieve only so much, and perhaps the message to emerge most strongly from this research is that it can leave processes essentially as they were - unchanged. To the extent that reorganisation of the NHS in 1974 was a re-jigging of administrative structures, and little else, attitudes have remained basically unchanged. In short, despite all the rhetoric, reorganisation has had a minimal impact on the cultural *milieu* of the NHS. Clearly, the architects of reform refrained from looking to see what *is* done within the Service, preferring instead to look at what *should* be done. Consequently, as Towell (56) has argued:

> 'left less than fully stated were the changes in power relationships required in order to achieve any radical impact on the prevailing distribution

of resources, both between different types of health provision and between different parts of the country. This understatement has partly reflected the technocratic bias in much thinking about these issues: the tendency to assume that better techniques of analysis and management would in themselves suffice to accomplish such changes'.

Organisational change, if it is to be introduced and managed successfully, probably needs to be incremental - although it is guided incrementalism, in the sense of there being a goal or set of goals, rather than disjointed incrementalism, in Braybrooke and Lindblom's secondary sense (57), that is involved. Planning and decision-making in the NHS, as in most organisations, are political processes but this has been insufficiently recognised or acted upon. A report (58) for the Royal Commission notes that 'the political aspect of planning was an example of the multiple perceptions of rationality that exist'. Practitioners and administrators, to cite two collective groups of decision actors, generally have different conceptions of what an ideal health service should be (59), and their differing views are not reconcilable through structural change alone. The report maintains that, in the end, 'planning statements come to represent the balance found between different concepts of rationality', and concludes that 'planning as a 'technology', a process of rationality, was not seen to have surmounted planning as an administrative or political exercise' (60).

Failure to view the NHS as a political system, that is, as a series of shifting coalitions of sectional groups, each with its own objectives, has led to a number of erroneous assumptions based on an image of the health service which stresses consensus and harmony. Concepts derived from scientific management were not so much determinants of the management model which emerged in 1974, as symptoms of a persistent belief in the unitary nature of organisational relationships in the NHS. If an attempt is made to look at processes (61), and to acknowledge the presence of a political dimension, perhaps, over time, not by frontal assault, which would be short-lived in its consequences and achieve little, but by adaptation and adjustment from within of existing arrangements in the light of experience, it will be possible to arrive at better and more relevant structure which are congruent with these processes (62). It is more than likely that 'undermining the foundations is just as effective a way of toppling a fortress as storming the ramparts' (63).

There are indications that the need 'to retain political realism' in decision processes is now being recognised (64). This research suggests that there is a need to go more quickly in this direction. Faith in the rational model of decision-making seems to be waning and, similarly, faith in macro-systems change imposed uniformly from the centre seems less fashionable after the management traumas of recent years (although, regrettably, the Government's latest proposals for reforming the NHS suggest that this may not be so). Hopefully, if anything has been learned from the reorganisation of the NHS it has been its potential for creating the illusion of change and for raising expectations which cannot be fulfilled. Unfortunately, the current reform proposals with their emphasis on creating the 'right' structure may repeat this error unless restraint is shown. Realisable proposals for change, as has been argued, must start with the current system, since structural upheaval, as this research suggests, would once again be likely to leave processes undisturbed. An attachment to improved administrative machinery can be a substitute for change - a ploy which serves to distract attention only temporarily from the real policy dilemmas that have to be tackled, and from the inescapable political choices that have to be confronted. There are dilemmas in health service administration to which there are no final, once-and-for-all solutions. The case study, in a modest way, has pointed to some of these, including the dual nature of the NHS, with its professional component and its administrative component expressing different demands and expectations, the resolution of which lies in continuous negotiation among participants.

The challenge over the coming years in the NHS will be the successful deployment of counter-pressures aimed at shifting the Service in the direction of priorities agreed upon through political discourse.

This has implications for all groups involved in the provision and administration of health care: for the way in which professionals are trained and remunerated (e.g. GPs), and whether the right professionals are being trained to look after the right patients (65); for the way in which those entrusted with the task of managing health services locally are trained in order to equip them to cope with 'the politics of process' (66); and, finally, for those responsible for overseeing the activities of managers and professionals - health authority members - whose present position in the NHS is weakest of all. Regrettably, neither the Royal Commission, as mentioned, nor the Government has addressed itself to this issue. Both have pronounced on the sources of membership of health authorities but equally, perhaps more, important is the ability of members to perform their tasks, an area which has been neglected by reformers. Whether in the NHS, local government or elsewhere, 'the moves to strengthen public scrutiny, control, initiative and participation have been cautious, reluctant and trivial in comparison with the growth of administrative power' (67). The ability of lay members in the NHS to exert influence on officers (or rather their inability - the case study showed how the involvement of members in the allocation of DF was notable for its almost total absence) needs to be given serious attention and ways found of giving them a meaningful role in priority-setting. After all, the NHS is a public service and matters involving resource-allocation and priority-setting are political concerns. Decisions to close down a hospital, or establish a health centre, are as politically relevant to the public as any other decisions about housing, education and so on which are taken by local councillors. Health planning and policy decisions are inescapably political in their impact on the quality of life. Therefore, accountability, by which is meant giving reasons for, and explanations of, what goes on, is of major importance. In the NHS it should mean an acceptance of the responsibility publicly to explain and justify policies, a willingness to welcome, rather than stifle, discussion of priorities and objectives, and an awareness of, and sensitivity to, public needs. Direct clashes of values should be directly resolved and not side-stepped 'with the aid of magic incantations' (68). True accountability may be more difficult to achieve in a complicated, interdependent age but this is no excuse for abandoning the attempt.

Notes and References

Chapter 1

1. This is especially evident in Scotland. For a comment, see Allen, C.H., 'The Study of Scottish Politics: A Bibliographical Sermon' in Drucker, N. and Drucker, H.M., eds., The Scottish Government Yearbook 1980, Paul Harris, Edinburgh, 1979, pp.11-41. Allen suggests that the Scottish political system is marked by six main features: centralisation, administrative primacy, exclusiveness, secrecy, corporatism and authoritarianism. These features, he argues, account in part for the 'slim material on policy-making' (p.13) in Scotland.
2. Ridley, F.F., 'Public Administration: Cause for Discontent', Public Administration, 50, Spring 1972, pp.70-1.
3. Stanyer, J., Understanding Local Government, Fontana, London, 1976.
4. See, for example, Boaden, N., Urban Policy-Making, Cambridge University Press, London, 1971; Lee, J.M. and Wood, B., The Scope of Local Initiative: a Study of Cheshire County Council, 1961-74, Martin Robertson, London, 1974; Dearlove, J., The Politics of Policy in Local Government, Cambridge University Press, London, 1973; Greenwood, R., Hinings, C.R. and Ranson, S., 'The Politics of the Budgetary Process in English Local Government', Political Studies, 25, 1, 1977, pp.25-47; Judge, K.,

Rationing Social Services, Heinemann, London, 1978, especially Chapter 5; Danziger, J.N., Making Budgets: Public Resource Allocation, Sage, London, 1979, especially Chapters 4 and 5. Also of note are Friend, J.K. and Jessop, W.N., Local Government and Strategic Choice, 2nd edition, Pergamon Press, Oxford, 1977, and Friend, J.K., Power, J. and Yewlett, C.J.L., Public Planning: the inter-corporate dimension, Tavistock, London, 1974. On education, see Kogan, M., The Politics of Education, Penguin, Harmondsworth, 1971; Kogan, M. County Hall: The Role of the Chief Education Officer, Penguin, Harmondsworth, 1974; Kogan, M. Educational Policy-Making, Allen and Unwin, London, 1975; Ribbins, P.M. and Brown, R.J., 'Policy Making in English Local Government: The Case of Secondary School Reorganization', Public Administration, 57, Summer 1979, pp.187-202. For analyses of policy-making in other areas of social policy, see Hall, P., Land, H., Parker, R. and Webb, A., Change, Choice and Conflict in Social Policy, Heinemann, London, 1975 and Donnison, D., Chapman, V,, Meacher, M., Sears, A. and Urwin, K., Social Policy and Administration Revisited, Allen and Unwin, London, 1975.

5. See Haywood, S.C., et al, 'The Outcome of NHS Reorganisation: Structural Change and Implementation of Social Policy', Public Administration Bulletin, No 31, December 1979; Brown, R.G.S., Reorganising the National Health Service: A Case Study of Administrative Change, Blackwell and Robertson, Oxford, 1979; Haywood, S.C. and Alaszewski, A., The NHS - Who Rules?, Croom Helm, London, forthcoming. For specifically Scottish studies, see Taylor, R., 'The local health system: an ethnography of interest-groups and decision-making', Social Science and Medicine, 11, 1977, pp.583-92; Taylor, R., 'The local health system: observations on the exercise of professional influence', Health and Social Service Journal, 21 July 1978, Centre Eight Papers, pp.B27-B32; Institute for Operational Research, Programme of Studies in Health Planning April 1974 - May 1976, IOR/883R, Edinburgh, May 1976.

6. See, for example, Davies, C., 'Professionals in Organisations: Some Preliminary Observations on Hospital Consultants', *Sociological Review*, *20*, 1972, pp.553-67; Freidson, E., *ed*., *The Professions and Their Prospects*, Sage, Beverly Mills, 1973; Green, S., 'Professional/Bureaucratic Conflict: The Case of the Medical Profession in the National Health Service', *Sociological Review*, *23*, 1975, pp.121-41.
7. For a comment, see Davis, A.G., 'An Unequivocal Change of Policy: Prevention Health and Medical Sociology', *Social Science and Medicine*, *13A*, March 1979, pp.129-37.
8. This is strongly advocated by Illsley, R., 'Promotion to observer status', *Social Science and Medicine*, *9*, 1975, pp.63-7; a similar point is made in Donnison, *et al*, *op.cit*.: 'Studies of administration tend to deal with the top or bottom levels of the structure: democratically elected bodies and their chief officers at one end: clients and those who serve them at the other. We neglect the levels between at our peril' (p.306). Support also comes from an SSRC advisory panel on health and health policy; see, Social Science Research Council, *Health and Health Policy: priorities for research*, report of an advisory panel to the Research Initiatives Board, London, June 1977.
9. See, for instance, Maddox, G.L., 'Muddling Through: Planning for Health Care in England', *Medical Care*, *9*, 5, September-October 1971, pp.439-48; Klein, R., 'Policy-Making in the National Health Service', *Political Studies*, *22*, March 1974, pp.1-14; Klein, R., 'Policy problems and policy perceptions in the National Health Service', *Policy and Politics*, *2*, 3, 1974, pp.219-36; Heidenheimer, A.J., Heclo, H.H. and Adams, C.T., *Comparative Public Policy*, Macmillan, London, 1976, Chapter 1; Allen, D., *Hospital Planning*, Pitman Medical, London, 1979.
10. Kogan, M., 'Book Review', *Political Quarterly*, *47*, 4, 1976, pp.490-91 and Kogan, M., 'Notes and Comments', *British Journal of Political Science*, *6*, 1976, pp.507-8. See also reply by Klein, R., *ibid*., p.509. On a similar point, see Glennerster, H.,

Social Service Budgets and Social Policy, Allen and Unwin, London, 1975, pp.258-59.

11. Watkin, B., 'Health care planning - comprehensive planning', Health and Social Service Journal, 20 September 1975, pp.2097-8 and 'Health care planning - participation', Health and Social Service Journal, 27 September 1975, pp.2169-70. In an attempt to remove some of the prevailing ignorance, the Royal Commission on the NHS commissioned a research team from Brunel University, under Professor Maurice Kogan, to study decision-making processes in the re-organised Service; see The working of the National Health Service, Research Paper Number 1, HMSO, London, 1978.
12. Stanyer, J. and Smith, B., Administering Britain, Fontana, London, 1976, p.266.
13. For a discussion of the Royal Commission's report and the Government's consultative papers, see Chapter 7.
14. Ample evidence exists to support this conclusion. Since the inception of the NHS, general policy statements have been issued by the DHSS indicating that increasing priority will be given to services for the mentally handicapped and mentally ill. Yet, as Heller, T., Restructuring the Health Service, Croom Helm, London, 1978, among others, has pointed out, these priorities 'have never been translated into an increased proportion of the budget spent on these particular services' (p.18). Townsend, P., 'Inequality in the Health Service', The Lancet, 15 June 1974, pp.1179-89, has documented some costs relating to different services in different types of hospital. He concluded that not only is less money spent per patient on medical care in the non-acute hospitals (i.e. services for the long stay and chronic ill, mentally ill and mentally handicapped), less is also spent on food, cleaning and domestic services; see also Radical Statistics Health Group, In Defence of the NHS, London, 1977. The DHSS acknowledges the persistence of these imbalances between different services but how committed it is, or rather how much authority it actually possesses, to do something about resolving them remains unclear. In the DHSS's consultative

document, Priorities for Health and Personal Social Services in England, HMSO, London, 1976, emphasis is placed on the elderly and on the handicapped, particularly the mentally disordered, as the client groups deserving of priority. A subsequent DHSS document, Priorities in the Health and Social Services: The Way Forward, HMSO, London, 1977, makes it clear that the main aim of health policy is 'to remedy past neglect of services, particularly those for the mentally ill and the mentally handicapped' (para. 1.14, p.6). However, there are more differences between these two priorities documents than similarities, and there is considerable scepticism concerning the DHSS's commitment to action. For instance, Brown, R.G.S., 'Accountability and control in the National Health Service', Health and Social Service Journal, 28 October 1977, Centre Eight Papers, pp.B9-B15, suggests that whereas the first priorities document 'gave a clear sense of direction about the need to alter priorities' within a given timescale, the later document 'was toned down from firm targets to hopeful aspirations' (p.B12). The Foreward of the later document makes it quite clear that 'significant and rapid changes in the desired directions (within the suggested time scale)' will not be possible (p.vii). The document proceeds to describe 'the general direction of service development ... but not the pace of change' (para. 1.5, p.2, emphasis added). Brown (ibid.) argues that 'the implications of the change from a prescriptive to a concessionary tone are clear enough', in particular the fact that what was proposed in the original document 'was not acceptable to the health authorities ...'. Furthermore, Brown, M., 'Priorities for health and personal social services', in Jones, K., ed., The Year Book of Social Policy in Britain 1976, Routledge and Kegan Paul, London, 1977, pp.21-34, notes that 'expenditure on the mentally ill and handicapped ... is actually projected to fall as a percentage of total expenditure' (p.29). Having referred to the 'long history of fine policy statements in this area of service and an equally long history of slow progress in implementing them', she quotes the conclusion of another commentator on social service affairs who was convinced that 'progress would be faster if we concentrated less on the nature of the problems themselves, and more on the constraints which impede the introduction of reforms' (ibid., emphasis added). For more recent evidence of the persistence of inequalities see Office of Health Economics, OHE Compendium of Health Statistics, 3rd edition, London, 1979, especially section 1, and Bosanquet, N. and Townsend, P., eds., Labour and Equality, Heinemann, London, 1980, Chapter 12.

15. See Chapter 2.
16. See, for example, Buxton, M.J. and Klein, R., 'Distribution of Hospital Provision: Policy Themes and Resource Variation', British Medical Journal, 8 February 1975, pp.345-48; Noyce, J., Snaith, A.H. and Trickey, A.J., 'Regional Variations in the Allocation of Financial Resources to the Community Health Services', The Lancet, 30 March 1974, pp.554-7; Rickard, J.H., 'Per capita expenditure of the English area health authorities', British Medical Journal, 31 January 1976, pp.299-300; Barnard, K. and Ham, C., 'The Reallocation of Resources', The Lancet, 26 June 1976, pp.1399-1400. The references cited in note 5 above are attempts to remedy the situation.
17. Heclo, H., 'Social Politics and Policy Impacts', in Holden Jr., M. and Dresang, D.L., eds., What Government Does, Sage, Beverly Hills, 1975, pp. 151-76; see also, Heclo, H., Modern Social Politics in Britain and Sweden, Yale University Press, London, 1975, pp.304-6.
18. Schon, D., Beyond the Stable State, Penguin, Harmondsworth, 1973.
19. Powell, E., Medicine and Politics, Pitman Medical, London, 1967.
20. Crossman, R.H.S., A Politician's View of Health Service Planning, University of Glasgow, 1972.
21. See Klein, 'Policy-Making in the National Health Service', op.cit.
22. For a comment on this see Mackenzie, W.J.M. Power and Responsibility in Health Care, Oxford University Press for Nuffield Provincial Hospitals Trust, London, 1979, especially Chapter 9.

23. Rhodes, R.A.W., 'Centre-Local Relations', in Appendix 6: The Relationship between Central and Local Government: Evidence and Commissioned Work, *Report of the Committee of Enquiry into Local Government Finance* (Layfield), Cmnd.6543, HMSO, London, 1976, p.187; see also, Rhodes, R.A.W., 'Research into Central-Local Relations in Britain: A Framework for Analysis', in SSRC, *Central-Local Government Relationships,* London, 1979, Appendix 1.
24. Confusion exists among social scientists as to whether decision-making and policy-making both have the same meaning, or whether there is a clear distinction between the two terms. For instance, Lowi, T., 'Decision-making vs. Policy-making: towards an antidote for technocracy', *Public Administration Review*, *30*, No.3, May/June 1970, pp.314-325, objects to the two terms being used interchangeably, arguing that they have quite separate conceptual meanings. On the other hand, Brown, R.G.S., *The Management of Welfare*, Fontana, London, 1975, sees the two terms as being interrelated. He describes policy-making as a process of reaching strategic decisions which alter the character, volume, or distribution of the relevant services. Policy in the NHS is the outcome of participation with authorities and management teams. Brown's merging of the two terms is akin to the definition of decision-making adopted by Friend, J.K. and Jessop, W.N., *op.cit*., in their study of decision-making in local government. There is a close affinity between the two terms in those instances where strategic choices are being made. The case study is concerned with decisions which have a strategic impact in that they have a direct affect on the sorts of services provided by health boards. These decisions are examples of middle-range decision-making, i.e. decisions with policy implications. For further discussion of some of these semantical problems, see Heclo, *Modern Social Politics in Britain and Sweden*, *op.cit*., p.4.
25. Wildavsky, A., *The Politics of the Budgetary Process*, Little, Brown and Co., Boston, 1964.
26. *ibid*., pp.v and 5.
27. Dearlove, *op.cit*.

28. These are discussed in more detail in Hunter, David, J., *Decisions and Resources in the National Health Service in Scotland*, Ph.D. thesis, University of Edinburgh, 1979; see also, Hunter, D.J., 'Practice: decisions and resources in the National Health Service (Scotland)' in Boyd, K.M., *ed*., *The Ethics of Resource Allocation in Health Care*, Edinburgh University Press, Edinburgh, 1979, Appendix 2.

Chapter 2

1. See Albrow, M., *Bureaucracy*, Macmillan, London, 1973, for a concise summary of the various models of bureaucracy.
2. See Susser, M.W. and Watson, W., *Sociology in Medicine*, Oxford University Press, London, 1971, especially Chapter 7.
3. See, for instance, Klein, R., 'Accountability in the NHS', *Political Quarterly*, *42*, 1971, pp.364-74; Klein, R., 'NHS: After Reorganisation', *Political Quarterly*, *44*, 1973, pp.316-28; Klein, R., 'An Anatomy of the NHS', *New Society*, 28 June 1973, pp.739-41; *New Society*, 'Guide to the new NHS', 28 February 1974, pp.514-17; Cooper, M.H., 'Rationing health', *New Society*, 18 April 1974, pp.131-2; Cooper, M.H., 'Rationing and Financing Health Care Resources', in Reekie, W.D. and Hunt, N.C., *eds*., *Management in the Social and Safety Services*, Tavistock, London, 1974, pp.11-34; Cooper, M.H., *Rationing Health Care*, Croom Helm, London, 1975; Brown, R.G.S., *The Management of Welfare*, Fontana, London, 1975; Culyer, A.J., 'Health: the social cost of doctors' discretion', *New Society*, 27 February 1975, pp.517-19; Culyer, A.J., *Need and the NHS: Economics and Social Choice*, Martin Robertson, London, 1976.
4. Freidson, E., *Professional Dominance*, Atherton Press, New York, 1970; Freidson, E., *Profession of Medicine*, Dodd, Mead and Co., New York, 1970.
5. Rowbottom, R., *et al*, *Hospital Organisation*, Heinemann, London, 1973, p.73.
6. Johnson, T.J., *Professions and Power*, Macmillan, London, 1972, pp.41-86.
7. *ibid*., p.57.

8. Cooper, 'Rationing health', *op.cit.*, p.18.
9. SHHD, *Organisation of Medical Work in the Hospital Service in Scotland* (Brotherston), HMSO, Edinburgh, 1967; SHHD, *Doctors in an Integrated Health Service*, HMSO, Edinburgh, 1971; SHHD, *The Organisation of a Medical Advisory Structure*, HMSO, Edinburgh, 1973.
10. See Foot, M., *Aneurin Bevan 1945-60*, vol.2, Paladin, London, 1973.
11. Armstrong, D., 'The Decline of the Medical Hegemony: A Review of Government Reports during the National Health Service', *Social Science and Medicine*, *10*, 1976, pp.157-63. See also, Martin, M., *Colleagues or Competitors?*, Occasional Papers on Social Administration No.31, Bell, London, 1969; McGlew, T. and Robertson, A., 'Social Change and the Shifting Boundaries of Discretion in Medicine', unpublished paper presented to SSRC Workshop on Discretion, Cambridge, July 1979.
12. McKinsey and Company, *Realizing the Promise of a National Health Service*, submission by team from McKinsey led by Banham, J. to the Royal Commission on the NHS, January 1977, para.3, p.9.
13. *ibid*.
14. See Davies, C., 'Hospital Consultants and Collective Action', amended draft of a paper presented to the BSA Medical Sociology Conference, York, November 1973.
15. The English equivalent of the Brotherston system in Scotland: see note 9 above.
16. See further, Hunter, David J., 'Patterns of Organisation for Health: A Systems Overview of the National Health Service in the United Kingdom', unpublished paper presented to SSRC Workshop on the Comparative Study of the Social Services in the United Kingdom, Edinburgh, September 1979. See also, Kellas, J.G., *The Scottish Political System*, 2nd edition, Cambridge University Press, London, 1975.
17. In an international context, growth of health care expenditure has been slower (it is presently falling) in the UK than elsewhere, as a percentage of GNP. For example, in the United States national expenditure on health services in 1977 represented almost 9% of GNP, whereas in the UK the comparable

figure was just under 5.5%. It has been estimated by McKinsey and Co that on present trends, US expenditure could easily exceed 15% of GNP in 20 years' time. In their evidence to the Royal Commission on the NHS, McKinsey and Co., op.cit., pointed out that 'there is ample evidence that, left to market forces, the cost of health care will escalate rapidly' (para.3, p.1.5).

18. Klein, R., 'Policy-making in the NHS', Political Studies, 22, March 1974, pp.1-14.
19. SHHD, The NHS and the Community in Scotland, HMSO, Edinburgh, 1974, para.21, p.6.
20. See Donald, B.L., 'Volunteers Retained as Managers: NHS Reorganisation Changes Authority Members' Role', Public Administration, 54, Autumn, 1975, p.303. See also, Hunter, David J., Decisions and Resources in the National Health Service in Scotland, Ph.D. thesis, University of Edinburgh, 1979, especially Chapter 7.
21. See SHHD Circulars HSR (72) C3, p.3 and HSR (73) C7.
22. SHHD Circular HSR (73) C7, p.2.
23. SHHD Circular HSR (72) C3, p.5.
24. Institute of Health Service Administrators (IHSA), The Role of Unit and Sector Administrators in the National Health Service, report of a joint working party, London, 1976, p.v.
25. SHHD, Reorganisation of the Scottish Health Services, Cmnd.4734, HMSO, London, 1971, para.55, p.17.
26. SHHD Circular HSR (72) C3.
27. DHSS, Guide to Planning in the NHS, HMSO, London, 1975.
28. There are mixed views among Scottish Health Service administrators over the advantages/disadvantages of a line management relationship between area officers and district officers. A review of the management of the reorganised NHS, undertaken by a working party of the Association of Chief Administrators of Health Authorities in December 1975, discovered no evidence of very strong advocacy for the area and district line relationship in Scotland, although some respondents supported it, saying that it ensured uniformity within the area, protected the smaller

districts and might improve effectiveness. The report continued, 'Both Area and District Administrators mentioned difficulties resulting from the line relationship including the danger of the District's collective responsibilities being disrupted by an individual officer at Area level, of clinicians 'going to the top' and by-passing the District, of District officers needing to check with their superiors and report back and there were suggestions that this all caused delays' (section 7.3, para.3, p.36).

29. SHHD, Administrative Practice of Hospital Boards in Scotland (Farquharson-Lang), HMSO, Edinburgh, 1966, para.30, p.13.
30. SHHD Circular HSR (72) C3.
31. The recommendations of the Farquharson-Lang Committee in 1966 were along very similar lines to those which emerged with reorganisation, but it is not possible to state to what extent the former RHBs had implemented the proposals contained in the Farquharson-Lang report. However, it took re-organisation to introduce the necessary structural and organisational changes to facilitate the adoption of a management system which separated management from community representation and which attempted to give board members a more strategic policy-making role to perform. Nevertheless, Farquharson-Lang was a significant event as far as the Scottish Health Service is concerned since the report did create a climate in which the final re-organisation proposals evolved.
32. Brown, op.cit., p.203.
33. See, for example, Brown, R.G.S., The Administrative Process in Britain, Allen and Unwin, London 1970; Hill, M.J., The Sociology of Public Administration, Weidenfeld and Nicholson, London 1972; Keeling, D., Management in Government, Allen and Unwin, London 1972; Self, P., Administrative Theories and Politics, second edition, Allen and Unwin, London 1977; Stanyer, J. and Smith, B., Administering Britain, Fontana, London 1976.
34. Quoted in Hill, op.cit., p.203.
35. SHHD Circular HSR (72) C3.
36. See further Chapter 7.
37. Stanyer and Smith, op.cit., p.191.

38. Heclo, H., 'The Councillor's Job', <u>Public Administration</u>, <u>47</u>, 1969, pp.185-202; see also, Hill, op.cit., Chapters 10 and 11.
39. Boddy, D., 'An Experiment in the Long-Term Planning of Health Services', <u>Public Administration</u>, <u>57</u>, Summer 1979, p.164.
40. SHHD, Scottish Health Service Planning Council, <u>Report for 1974</u>, HMSO, Edinburgh 1975.
41. See Wiseman, C., 'Strategic Planning in the Scottish NHS - A Mixed-Scanning Approach', <u>Long Range Planning</u>, April 1979; also, Wiseman, C., 'Selection of Major Planning Issues', <u>Policy Sciences</u>, <u>9</u>, 1978.
42. SHHD, <u>The Health Service in Scotland: The Way Ahead</u>, HMSO, Edinburgh, 1976.
43. SHHD, 'The New Influences on Decision-Making in the Reorganised Health Service', draft of a talk given by the Secretary to Health Services Conference, unpublished, May 1973.
44. SHHD, <u>The Organisation of a Medical Advisory Service</u>, <u>op.cit</u>., para.3.4, p.6.
45. Levitt, R., <u>The Reorganised National Health Service</u>, Croom Helm, London, 1976, p.181.
46. SHHD, <u>Health Services in Scotland: Report for 1977</u>, Cmnd.7237, HMSO, Edinburgh, 1978, para.8.4, p.44.
47. See note 32 above, p.156.
48. DHSS, <u>Sharing Resources for Health in England</u>: report of the resource allocation working party (RAWP), HMSO, London, 1976; SHHD, <u>Scottish Health Authorities Revenue Equalisation</u> (<u>SHARE</u>): report of the working party on resource allocation, HMSO, Edinburgh, 1977.
49. Gentle, P.H. and Forsythe, J.M., 'Revenue Allocation in the Reorganised NHS', <u>British Medical Journal</u>, <u>3</u>, 9 August 1975, pp.382-4.
50. SHHD, <u>Interim Report</u>: working party on revenue resource allocation, September 1976, para.9, Appendix 2 of <u>SHARE</u>, <u>op.cit</u>., p.54.
51. See <u>The Guardian</u>, 7 September 1977 for a good example of these tensions at work. Money (about £5 million) allocated by the DHSS specifically to establish regional secure units in psychiatric hospitals was used by some RHAs 'to shore up their general revenue accounts and, in one case, to offset revenue overspending'. One MP requested

an inquiry into the way in which 'money allocated nationally for a nationally-determined priority has been misapplied by these authorities'. The DHSS emphasised that 'although regions have been told to keep the special funds available to run secure units, there is no prohibition on their using the money for other purposes in the meantime'. It would require an Act of Parliament to enable the DHSS to ensure that health authorities spent the money according to its wishes and not according to the authorities' own priorities.

52. See note 50 above.
53. Steele, R. and Mooney, G., 'SHARE: the case for equity in health care', The Scotsman, 13 September 1977.
54. Friend, J., 'Inter-Organisational Decision-Making in the Provision of Local Community Services: ...', IOR/876, Institute for Operational Research, October 1975, pp.14-5.
55. Rhodes, R.A.W., 'Research into Central-Local Relations in Britain: A Framework for Analysis', in SSRC, Central-Local Government Relationships, London, 1979, Appendix 1, p.17.
56. ibid.
57. Lee, K., 'Public Expenditure, Planning and Local Democracy', in Barnard, K. and Lee, K., eds., Conflicts in the National Health Service, Croom Helm, London, 1977, p.219.

Chapter 3

1. See, in particular, Bachrach, P. and Baratz, M.S., 'The Two Faces of Power', American Political Science Review, 56, 1962, pp.947-52; 'Decisions and Non-decisions: An Analytical Framework', American Political Science Review, 57, 1963, pp.641-51; Power and Poverty, Oxford University Press, New York, 1970.
2. Dubin, R., 'Stability of Human Organisation', in Haire, M., ed., Modern Organisation Theory, Wiley and Sons, Chicago, 1959, p.218.
3. Dearlove, J., The Politics of Policy in Local Government, Cambridge University Press, Cambridge, 1973. See also excerpts from Dearlove, op.cit., in Castles, F.G., et al, eds., Decisions,

Organisations and Society, second edition, Penguin, Harmondsworth, 1976, pp.96-128.

4. Bachrach and Baratz, op.cit.
5. Parry, G. and Morriss, P., 'When is a Decision not a Decision?', in Crewe I., ed., British Political Sociology Yearbook, Vol.1, Croom Helm, London, 1974, p.324.
6. Klein, R., in a review of Nicholson, M., The System, in The Observer, 24 September 1967 and cited in Levin, P.H., 'On Decisions and Decision Making', Public Administration, 50, 1972, p.41.
7. See, for example, Sharkansky, I., The Routines of Politics, Van Nostrand Reinhold, New York, 1970; also, Edwards III, George C. and Sharkansky, I., The Policy Predicament, Freeman, San Francisco, 1978.
8. Parry and Morriss, op.cit., p.334.
9. See note 7 above.
10. Lukes, S., Power, Macmillan, London, 1974.
11. ibid., p.19. Barber, J.D., Power in Committees, Rand McNally and Co, Chicago, 1966, p.5, argues that power is 'a topic of some interest and much frustrating complexity for political scientists'. Barber's study, which is of some relevance to the case study, analyses power in committees by examining the process of making a budget and by considering the values and perceptions which committee members bring to bear on decision-making. The case study presented in the present research is not about power as such. It is about decision-making and the calculations and strategies involved in allocating resources in a particular area of resource-allocation. However, it is not possible to examine who gets what and why without considering the power implications of these decisions. Apart from the possible exercise of power within a committee itself, power may also lie outside it but still have an impact on the decisions which are made (cf. Lukes, op.cit.). Barber discusses the problems surrounding power analysis, including the dilemma of defining the term. He concludes that no single research project can span the entire range of possible definitions of power. The only way out of the confusion is to investigate those aspects

considered to be significant, or possibly significant, in a particular research setting. For Barber, the focus of his power analysis was on the operative distribution of power - the practical relations of conflict and compromise - as seen through the eyes of the participants. This approach is in line with the phenomenological method which underlies the case study to some degree (see note 112 below). 'Power ... is contextual in character. It is not an isolated, temporary phenomenon abstracted from the flow of life ...' (Barber, op.cit., p.47). Arguments about power are posed within a framework of concepts - time, knowledge, organisation and values. These concepts are elements of the framework which provides the present case study with its focus and means of structuring the field to be observed. Therefore, power is studied in a political sense - it is shaped and distributed by participants in accordance with certain shared values and perceptions (ibid., p.72). Barber maintains that the advantage of this method is that it gets at values and perceptions which are operative, in that they are linked by the respondents themselves to the practical problems and solutions which they develop.

12. Lukes, op.cit., p.23.
13. Heclo, H., 'Social Politics and Policy Impacts', in Holden Jr., M. and Dresang, D.L., eds., What Government Does, Sage, Beverly Hills, 1975, pp.151-176.
14. ibid., p.152.
15. See Chapter 2.
16. Maxwell, R., 'An Introduction', Paine, L., ed., The Health Service Administrator: Innovator or Catalyst?, King Edward's Hospital Fund for London, London, 1978, pp.101-2.
17. Mitchell, R., 'Resources in Scottish Health Services', in Paine, op.cit., p.119.
18. Heclo, 'Social Politics and Policy Impacts', op. cit. See also, Heclo, H., Modern Social Politics in Britain and Sweden, Yale University Press, London, 1974, pp.304-305.
19. Heclo, 'Social Politics and Policy Impacts', op. cit., p.153.

20. Rivlin, A., 'Obstacles to Social Progress: Why Can't We Get Things Done', Washington Post, 22 July 1971 and cited in Rein, M., Social Science and Public Policy, Penguin, Harmondsworth, 1976, p.57.
21. See Chapter 1.
22. Self, P., Administrative Theories and Politics, second edition, Allen and Unwin, London, 1977, p.4.
23. See Chapter 2.
24. See Chapter 2.
25. See Chapter 5.
26. Self, op.cit., p.8.
27. ibid.
28. See Chapter 7.
29. For succinct summaries of the theories of the principal thinkers of this school, see Kempner, A.T. and Wills, G., eds., Management Thinkers, Penguin, Harmondsworth, 1978, pp.73-96, 108-39. See also, March, J.G. and Simon, H.A., Organisations, Wiley and Sons, New York, 1958, Chapter 2.
30. Self, op.cit., pp.7-8.
31. See Edwards III and Sharkansky, op.cit., p.273.
32. ibid., p.274.
33. See Morris, J.N., 'Tomorrow's Community Physician' in Gatherer, A. and Warren, M.D., eds., Management and the Health Services, Pergamon Press, Oxford, 1971, pp.151-66. Some observers have suggested that there has been a preoccupation with management techniques as reflected in the job specifications and training of CMSs. There have been criticisms of the way in which the specialty has evolved since reorganisation. Symptomatic of deeper structural issues has been mounting confusion within the specialty over the nature of its precise function. Towell, D., 'Making Re-organisation Work: Challenges and Dilemmas in the Development of Community Medicine', in Barnard, K. and Lee, K., eds., Conflicts in the National Health Service, Croom Helm, London, 1977, pp.167-88, provides valuable insights into some of these problems. See also, Heller, T., Restructuring the Health Service, Croom Helm, London, 1978, pp.78-9, and the Unit for the Study of Health Policy,

Rethinking Community Medicine, London, June 1979.

34. Such a distinction has been made by Patrick Jenkin, at the time of writing Secretary of State for Social Services; see Health and Social Service Journal, 8 June 1979, p.683.
35. See Chapter 2.
36. Allison, G.T., Essence of Decision, Little, Brown, Boston, 1971.
37. See Greenwood, R., et al, 'The Politics of the Budgetary Process in English Local Government' Political Studies, 25, 1, 1977, p.38.
38. See Chapter 2.
39. Dimmock, S. and Barnard, K., 'Relationships and Communications' in Raybould, E., ed., A Guide for Nurse Managers, Blackwell, Oxford, 1977, pp.81-103.
40. ibid., pp.98-9.
41. ibid., p.102.
42. These include: Lindblom, C.E., 'The Science of "Muddling Through"', Public Administration Review, 19, 1959, pp.79-88; 'Contexts for Change and Strategy: a Reply', Public Administration Review, 24, 1964, pp.157-8; The Policy-Making Process, Prentice-Hall, New Jersey 1968; with Braybrooke, D., A Strategy of Decision, Free Press, New York, 1963.
43. The attempt to procure savings in the two health boards was illustrative of the primary meaning of 'disjointed'; see Chapters 5 and 6 for other instances too.
44. Braybrooke and Lindblom, op.cit., p.106.
45. See March and Simon, op.cit., pp.169-71.
46. Allison, op.cit.
47. Allison, G.T. and Halperin, M.H., 'Bureaucratic Politics', World Politics, 24, Spring 1972; see also Allison, op.cit., p.272.
48. Dimmock and Barnard, op.cit., p.85.
49. ibid., p.86.
50. Wheaton, cited in Alden, J. and Morgan, R., Regional Planning: A Comprehensive View, Heath and Reach, Leighton Buzzard, 1974, p.173.
51. See, for example, Wildavsky, A., The Politics of the Budgetary Process, Little, Brown, Boston, 1964; Crecine, J.P., Governmental Problem-Solving, Rand McNally and Co, Chicago, 1969.
52. Ball, op.cit.

53. Allison, op.cit.
54. Wildavsky, op.cit.
55. See Chapter 6.
56. March and Simon, op.cit., pp.137-42.
57. Greenwood et al, op.cit.
58. ibid., p.27.
59. Cornford, J.P., 'Review Article: The Illusion of Decision', British Journal of Political Science, 4, 1974, pp.238-9.
60. ibid., p.239.
61. Ruggie, J.C., 'Complexity, Planning, and Public Order', in La Porte, T., ed., Organised Social Complexity, Princeton University Press, New Jersey, 1975, pp.134-5.
62. The role of fashion in social policy-making should not be under-estimated. Higgins, J., The Poverty Business: Britain and America, Blackwell/Martin Robertson, London 1978, in her account of poverty policies over the last decade or so, draws attention to the importance of fashion in the adoption of a social engineering approach to change. Klein, R., 'Reorganisation: what went wrong', New Society, 22 September 1977, p.593, notes that 'the intellectual fashions which led to the wave of reorganisation in the 1960s and 1970s have been displaced by a new set of fashions'. There is now less enthusiasm for social engineering and rational, synoptic solutions to social problems. There is, as Self (op.cit.) and others have noted, a resurgence of political as against administrative values. See also Schon, D., Beyond the Stable State, Penguin, Harmondsworth, 1973, for a discussion of his notion of 'ideas in good currency', pp.115ff.
63. Greenwood et al, op.cit., p.27.
64. Mitchell, op.cit., p.113.
65. Judge, K., Rationing Social Services, Heinemann, London 1978.
66. ibid., pp.107-8.
67. Danziger, J.N., 'Assessing Incrementalism in British Municipal Budgeting', British Journal of Political Science, 6, 1976, pp.335-350; see also, Danziger, J.N., Making Budgets: Public Resource Allocation, Sage, London 1979.
68. Lukes, op.cit., pp.24-5.
69. Cornford, op.cit., p.239.

70. Klein, R., 'Policy-making in the National Health Service', Political Studies, 20, No.1, 1974, pp.1-14; also, Klein, R., 'Policy Problems and Perceptions in the National Health Service', Policy and Politics, 2, 1974, pp.219-236.
71. Rein, op.cit.
72. ibid., p.260.
73. ibid., p.261.
74. Dror, Y., Public Policy-Making Re-examined, Leonard Hill Books, Aylesbury, 1973.
75. See Chapter 1, note 14.
76. Klein, 'Policy Problems and Perceptions in the NHS', op.cit.
77. DHSS, Management Arrangements for the Reorganised National Health Service, HMSO, London, 1972, para.1.5, e, p.10.
78. Cornford, op.cit., p.236.
79. ibid.
80. ibid.
81. Danziger, 'Assessing Incrementalism in British Municipal Budgeting', op.cit.
82. ibid., p.110.
83. ibid.
84. ibid., p.111.
85. ibid., p.112.
86. See Heclo, H. and Wildavsky, A., The Private Government of Public Money, Macmillan, London, 1974, where the authors' observations of the Public Expenditure Survey Committee (PESC) tend to confirm the paradox between the employment of management techniques and their reinforcement, or encouragement, of incrementalism. 'PESC has enshrined incrementalism with a vengeance' (p.238). 'Incrementalism has been reinforced through PESC by making each department more conscious of its own fair share of the total and more aware of other departments' departures from the expected rate of increase. In this sense, PESC has increased openness by reducing the scope for back-stairs deals between Treasury and spending ministers. Vastly increasing a programme of switching priorities must be registered ... in the open' (p.239). PESC has operated to make it 'more difficult to depart from the historical base' (p.238).

87. See Chapter 7.
88. Allison, op.cit.
89. March and Simon, op.cit., p.139.
90. Cornford, op.cit., p.237.
91. ibid.
92. Dror, op.cit.
93. Carrier, J. and Kendall, I., 'Social policy and social change - explanations of the development of social policy', Journal of Social Policy, 2, 1973, pp.209-24. The authors' approach is based on a phenomenological perspective, that is, one that 'reinstates human experience in its place as the primary datum about the world and it describes this experience by turning and returning to the intentional features of experience', Luckman, T., ed., Phenomenology and Sociology, Penguin, Harmondsworth, 1978, p.8. Carrier and Kendall argue that a phenomenological approach 'is based on the acceptance of the presence of "multiple realities"', therefore, 'an adequate account of policy development might be considered as one which presents as systematically as possible the participants' explanations of "why things happened as they did" and "why certain decisions were taken"' (p.221). The 'assumptive world' of decision-makers has been discussed by Young, K., '"Values" in the Policy Process', Policy and Politics, 5, 1977, pp.1-22.
94. Silverman, D. in Filmer, P., et al, New Directions in Sociological Theory, Collier-Macmillan, London, 1972, p.189 and cited in Carrier and Kendall, op. cit., p.222.
95. Klein, 'Policy problems and perceptions in the NHS', op.cit., p.219.
96. Rein, op.cit., p.77.
97. ibid.
98. Barnard, C.I., The Functions of the Executive, Cambridge, Massachusetts, 1966, pp.192-3.
99. Hall, P., et al, Change, Choice and Conflict in Social Policy, Heinemann, London, 1975, p.17.
100. Donnison, D., et al, Social Policy and Administration Revisited, Allen and Unwin, London, 1975, p.46.
101. For a full discussion of this point, see Hunter, David J., Decisions and Resources in the National

Health Service in Scotland, Ph.D. thesis, University of Edinburgh, 1979, Chapter 8.

102. See further Chapter 7.

103. A complete list of interviews is given at Appendix 1.

104. See further Chapters 5 and 6.

Chapter 4

1. There was no ready explanation for this difference, other than the fact that, as noted later in the chapter, district B was of the opinion that its hospital services were substandard in comparison with those in district A.
2. For further discussion of this point see Chapter 7.
3. Programme planning groups (or committees) were not studied in Alpha and Beta since they were in the process of being set up. Basically, the groups are involved in problem-solving from a multi-disciplinary perspective. See Boddy, D., 'An Experiment in the Long-Term Planning of Health Care Services', Public Administration, 57, Summer 1979, pp.159-71.
4. This point is developed in Chapter 6.
5. See further Chapter 6.
6. SHHD, Health Service Reorganisation Scotland, HSR (72) C1 - HSR (74) C12.
7. For further discussion of this point, see Hunter, David, J., Decisions and Resources in the NHS in Scotland, Ph.D. thesis, University of Edinburgh, 1979, Chapter 7.
8. See, for example, Pressman, J.L. and Wildavsky, A., Implementation, University of California Press, Berkeley, 1973; Hood, C.C., The Limits of Administration, Wiley and Sons, London, 1976.

Chapter 5

1. This point is explored further in Chapter 6.
2. NHS Circular No.1976 (GEN) 16, para.2, p.1.
3. ibid., para.11, p.3.
4. ibid., para.13, p.4.
5. The argument over costs and savings in preventive medicine is a complex one. For instance, increasing

expenditure on prevention tenfold will not lead to an equivalent saving on curative services. Indeed, it is likely to increase the demand on them. Effective prevention is likely only to delay expenditure. Therefore, investment in prevention cannot be justified on simple economic grounds despite the fact that many pronouncements on the subject emphasise this aspect. In the present example, fluoridation and preventive dentistry, such a policy would be likely to increase demand for conservative dentistry which would require an injection of resources.

6. This argument needs to be qualified. According to an editorial in The Hospital and Health Services Review, 72, No.5, May 1976, pp.147-8, 'It is more efficient to process patients more quickly but more intensive activity is also more expensive. If the result is more patients treated in the same beds rather than the same patients treated in fewer beds, costs will rise'. This is the inevitable outcome of the operation of supply and demand in health care and requires caution about the efficacy of day admissions, shorter treatment and so on.

7. According to Heller, T., Restructuring the Health Service, Croom Helm, London, 1978, lack of appropriate data is hampering the tasks of those engaged in community medicine. He argues that 'the NHS collects information on the state of the service rather than on the illness behaviour or health of the community' (p.78).

8. SHHD, The Health Service in Scotland: The Way Ahead, HMSO, Edinburgh 1976. All the priorities documents, including The Way Ahead, have been criticised for (a) being rather weak in their statements of intent in redressing the imbalances within the NHS; and (b) for some of the value judgements which underlie their conclusions concerning the need to shift resources from the hospital service to the community care service. For example, certain assumptions about the advantages of community care are stated when there exists little data to support them. In para.4.4, p.16, in The Way Ahead, it is stated 'that Boards should continue to accord priority to the

provision of health centres as the most effective means of promoting the development of primary care'. There is no reference to the possible disadvantages of health centres, particularly their location and access. Much of what is said in the documents about the need for preventive health remains at the level of pure rhetoric. Heller notes that 'although <u>Priorities for Health</u> accepts that preventive efforts and health education should become part of the general work of all sections of the caring services, and in particular of the primary care service, the section on preventive health might easily be criticised as pure rhetoric in the absence of any real diversion of funds to this sector' (p.97). For further criticisms of the English priorities document, see <u>Whose Priorities?</u>, Pamphlet 1, Radical Statistics Health Group, London, 1976, See also Chapter 1, note 2.

9. SHHD, <u>op.cit.</u>, para.1.3, p.7.
10. <u>ibid</u>., para.3.2, p.12.
11. <u>ibid</u>., para.3.13, p.14.
12. <u>ibid</u>., para.4, p.4.
13. See discussion of this relationship in Chapter 2; see also Chapter 6.
14. See notes 5 and 6 above.
15. In Grampian Health Board, the introduction of programme budgeting (PB) at the same time as the priorities memorandum appeared to give an added impetus to members' involvement in board affairs. For an account of PB see Mooney, G., 'Programme budgeting in an area health board', <u>The Hospital and Health Services Review</u>, <u>73</u>, No.11, November 1977, pp.379-384. PB is a tool of policy-making and not a substitute for the exercise of judgement. At best, PB will better inform this judgement by presenting data in such a way that it is possible to identify trends in spending on particular programmes of care. In this way it can provide ammunition for those, like health authority members, who at present experience extreme difficulty in performing a useful role in planning services (see Chapter 7). PB at local level is developing rapidly in Scotland. In contrast, there has been little activity in England in this field

(see Lee, K. and Mills, A., 'The contribution of economics to health service planning', Health and Social Service Journal, 8 February 1979, Centre Eight Papers, p.C38).

16. The report was the outcome of nearly 18 months' work. The feeling in Beta was that policies could not be established in the absence of detailed knowledge of existing services in the area. A working party (10 members, half of whom were board members) was set up shortly after reorganisation with the following terms of reference: 'Report to the Board on the provision of existing resources and facilities within the area of (Beta) and as far as possible to assess the health needs of the population and determine objectives to meet these needs'.

Chapter 6

1. Wildavsky, A., The Politics of the Budgetary Process, Little, Brown, Boston, 1964, pp.11ff.
2. Towell, D., 'Making Reorganisation Work: Challenges and Dilemmas in the Development of Community Medicine', in Barnard, K. and Lee, K., eds., Conflicts in the National Health Service, Croom Helm, London, 1977, p.176.
3. For instance, Klein, R., ed., Social Policy and Public Expenditure 1975: Inflation and Priorities, Centre for Studies in Social Policy/ Macmillan, London, 1975, p.89, argues that improving the NHS by adding to its manpower is only one possible policy option. Improving the use made of the NHS's manpower (while freezing or even reducing numbers) is another policy option. Klein suggests that more efficient use could be made of ancillary workers instead of constantly increasing their numbers. In the case of nursing and midwifery resources, Klein believes that their misallocation and maldistribution are more of a problem than shortages through failure to recruit or retain. Klein concedes, however, that it is the number of consultants which tends to determine the level of supporting staff needed and the demand for resources generated.

4. See Chapter 3.
5. Mitchell, R., 'The first year of the reorganised Scottish Health Service; a personal viewpoint', *The Hospital and Health Service Review*, *71*, No.5, 1975, p.161.
6. Brown, R.G.S., *et al*, *New Bottles: Old Wine*?, Institute for Health Studies, University of Hull, September 1975, p.24.
7. For a discussion of the arguments both for and against merging health and local authorities, see Hunter, David J., *Decisions and Resources in the National Health Service in Scotland*, Ph.D. thesis, University of Edinburgh, 1979, Chapter 3.
8. See, for example, SHHD/SED, *A Better Life: report on services for the mentally handicapped in Scotland*, HMSO, Edinburgh, 1979, pp.25-7. However, the Mitchell report (SHHD, *Working Party on Relationships between Health Boards and Local Authorities - Report*, HMSO, Edinburgh, 1977) did not consider that changes were required to the financial arrangements between health boards and local authorities. The working party favoured the creation of Joint Liaison Committees as a means of promoting co-operation.
9. For a view on this, see DHSS, *Making Whitley Work: a review of the operation of the NHS Whitley Council System (McCarthy)*, London, 1976, especially Chapter 7, pp.68-83.
10. See NHS Circular No 1976 (GEN) 16.
11. Klein, *op.cit*.
12. See Chapter 2; also, Armstrong, D., 'The Decline of the Medical Hegemony: ...', *Social Science and Medicine*, *10*, No.3/4, 1976, pp.157-163; Manson, T., 'Management, the Professions and the Unions ...', in Stacy, M., *et al*, *eds*., *Health and the Division of Labour*, Croom Helm, London, 1976.
13. A similar conclusion is reached by Taylor, R., 'The local health system: observations on the exercise of professional influence', *Health and Social Service Journal*, 21 July 1978, Centre Eight Papers, p.B32, who refers to 'waving the shroud' as 'that fail-safe professional tactic'.
14. Wildavsky, *op.cit*., pp.10-11.

15. Edwards III, G.C., and Sharkansky, I., The Policy Predicament, Freeman, San Francisco, 1978, p.263.
16. ibid., p.12.
17. In the questionnaire circulated to 10 health boards, boards were asked to comment on three allocation strategies: (i) fair shares; (ii) who will it hurt least?; and (iii) who has done all right so far?. It was a difficult question to answer and some responses seemed evasive. However, three boards reported that the strategies did play a part in their allocations; three reported that the strategies were not applicable, and four replied in equivocal terms suggesting that the strategies might, on occasion, have been deployed. See Hunter, op.cit., pp.603-4 for a full analysis.
18. Hunter, op.cit., Chapter 13.
19. See, for example, Abrams, P., 'Community Care: Some Research Problems and Priorities', in Barnes, J. and Connelly, N., eds., Social Care Research, Policy Studies Institute/DHSS, London, 1978, pp.78-9.
20. SHHD, Health Services in Scotland, Report for 1975, Cmnd.6506, HMSO, Edinburgh 1976, para.10.3, p.75; Report for 1976, Cmnd.6812, HMSO, Edinburgh 1977, para.9.3, p.66; Report for 1977, Cmnd.7237, HMSO, Edinburgh 1978, para.8.2, p.43; Report for 1978, Cmnd.76-7, HMSO, Edinburgh 1979, para.8.1, p.45.
21. For further discussion of this point, see correspondence in The Lancet: Constable, G.N., 'Decision Making in the NHS', 15 September 1979, p.587; reply by Hunter, David J., 'Decision Making in the NHS', 13 October 1979, p.802.
22. Mackenzie, W.J.M., Power and Responsibility in Health Care, Oxford University Press for the Nuffield Provincial Hospitals Trust, London, 1979, p.146.

Chapter 7

1. Royal Commission on the National Health Service, Report, Cmnd.7615, HMSO, London, July 1979. For a comment on the background to the setting up of the Commission, see Ryan, M., 'The Royal Commission on the NHS - Origins and Prospect', Social and Economic Administration, 11, Autumn 1977, pp.194-205.
2. DHSS, Patients First, HMSO, London, December 1979. For proposals which apply specifically to the Scottish Health Service, see SHHD, Structure and Management of the NHS in Scotland, HMSO, Edinburgh, 1979.
3. For a discussion of this concept, see Cooper, M.H., Rationing Health Care, Croom Helm, London, 1975, and Culyer, A.J., Need and the National Health Service, Martin Robertson, London, 1976.
4. Schultze, C., The Politics and Economics of Public Spending, The Brookings Institution, Washington, 1968.
5. Wildavsky, A., The Politics of the Budgetary Process, Little, Brown, Boston, 1964, pp.14-18
6. Braybrooke, D. and Lindblom, C.E., A Strategy of Decision, Free Press, New York, 1963.
7. Greenwood, R., 'The Local Authority Budgetary Process', in Booth, T.A., ed., Planning for Welfare, Blackwell and Robertson, Oxford, 1979, pp.93 ff.
8. Schon, D., Beyond the Stable State, Penguin, Harmondsworth, 1973, p.115.
9. The Royal Commission on the National Health Service, The Working of the National Health Service, Research Paper Number 1, HMSO, London, 1978, para 81, p.125.
10. Greenwood, op.cit.
11. See Chapter 3 above, note 86.
12. See note 9 above, para.74, p.123.
13. Lukes, S., Power, Macmillan, London, 1974. See also, Chapter 3 above.
14. Heclo, H., Modern Social Politics in Britain and Sweden, Yale University Press, London, 1974, p.305.
15. ibid., p.306.

16. Blandford, J., 'Appraising Quality and Effectiveness in Australia', in Paine, L., ed., The Health Service Administrator: Innovator or Catalyst?, King Edward's Hospital Fund for London, London, 1978, pp.165-6.
17. See, for instance, Boyd, K.M., ed., The Ethics of Resource Allocation in Health Care, Edinburgh University Press, Edinburgh, 1979, especially Chapter 2.
18. For a comprehensive study of LHCs see Bochel, D. and MacLaran, M., The Establishment and Development of Local Health Councils, Scottish Health Service Studies, 41, SHHD, Edinburgh, 1979.
19. See Hunter, David J., Decisions and Resources in the National Health Service in Scotland, unpublished Ph.D. thesis, University of Edinburgh, 1979, Chapter 7.
20. ibid.
21. Danziger, J.N., Making Budgets: Public Resource Allocation, Sage, London, 1978, p.225.
22. Mitchell, R., 'Resources in Scottish Health Services', in Paine, op.cit., p.115.
23. Gouldner, A.W., Patterns of Industrial Bureaucracy, Free Press, New York, 1964, p.28.
24. op.cit.
25. DHSS, op.cit.; SHHD, op.cit.; DHSS (Northern Ireland), Consultative Paper on the Structure and Management of Health and Personal Social Services in Northern Ireland, HMSO, Belfast, 1979.
26. House of Commons, Health Services Bill No. 98, HMSO, London, 1979.
27. Royal Commission on the NHS, op.cit., para.3.23, p.27.
28. ibid., p.297.
29. ibid., para.20.1, p.310.
30. ibid., para.20.33, p.321.
31. This is discussed further in Hunter, op.cit. See also, Haywood, S.C., 'More democracy for the NHS?', The Hospital and Health Services Review, 73, April 1977, pp.123-6.
32. Royal Commission on the NHS, Management of Financial Resources in the National Health Service, Research Paper Number 2, HMSO, London, 1978.
33. ibid., para.E2.1, p.199.

34. _ibid_., paras.E6.1 and E6.2, pp.202-3.
35. Royal Commission on the NHS, _op.cit_., para.21.53, p.348.
36. _ibid_., para.21.55, p.349.
37. McGlew, T. and Robertson, A., 'Social Change and the shifting Boundaries of Discretion in Medicine', unpublished paper presented to SSRC Workshop on Discretion, Cambridge, July 1979, pp.26 ff.
38. _ibid_.,
39. DHSS, _op.cit_., para.2, p.4.
40. The author is presently preparing a critique of the proposals. It is being produced by a small working group of health service administrators and academics interested in health policy based at the Outer Circle Policy Unit, London. The comments which follow are drawn, in part, from discussions within the group. See note 62 below.
41. See, for example, DHSS, _op.cit_., paras.8, 11, 16, 29, 37-40, pp.6, 7, 9, 15, 18-9.
42. This concept is taken from Lalonde, M., _A New Perspective on the Health of Canadians_, Ministry of National Health and Welfare, Canada, April 1974.
43. DHSS, _op.cit_., para.3, p.4.
44. For example, Office of Health and Economics, _Compendium of Health Statistics_, 3rd edition, London, 1979, especially Section 1; also, Bosanquet, N., 'Health', in Bosanquet, N. and Townsend, P., _eds_., _Labour and Equality_, Heinemann, London, 1980.
45. SHHD, _op.cit_., para.2, p.5.
46. _ibid_., para.12, p.8.
47. For an excellent account of these arising from NHS reorganisation in 1974, see Brown, R.G.S., _Reorganising the National Health Service: A Case Study of Administrative Change_, Blackwell and Robertson, Oxford, 1979, especially Chapter 10.
48. Hood, C.C., _The Limits of Administration_, Wiley and Sons, London, 1976, p.27.
49. See La Porte, T., _ed_., _Organised Social Complexity_, Princeton University Press, New Jersey, 1975.
50. Hoare, J., 'Bread and Games', _Hospital and Health Services Review_, _75_, October 1979, p.349.
51. Hood, _op.cit_., p.26.

52. Mant, A., The Rise and Fall of the British Manager, Macmillan, London, 1977, p.42.
53. DHSS, op.cit.
54. Hood, op.cit., p.27.
55. ibid.
56. Towell, D., 'Making Reorganisation Work: Challenges and Dilemmas in the Development of Community Medicine', in Barnard, K. and Lee, K., eds., Conflicts in the National Health Service, Croom Helm, London, 1977, p.168.
57. See discussion of incrementalism in Chapter 3.
58. See note 9 above, para.75, p.123.
59. See Tuckett, D., 'The Organization of Hospitals', in Tuckett, D., ed., An Introduction to Medical Sociology, Tavistock, London, 1976, pp.225-53.
60. See note 9 above, para.73, p.122. See also work of Scottish Institute for Operational Research, including Lind, G. and Wiseman, C., 'Setting Health Priorities: A Review of Concepts and Approaches', Journal of Social Policy, 7, 1978, pp.411-40; and Wiseman, C., 'Policy-Making for the Scottish Health Services at National Level', in Drucker, N. and Drucker, H.M., eds., The Scottish Government Yearbook 1980, Paul Harris, Edinburgh, 1979, pp.135-60.
61. For a discussion of process versus structure, see Olsen, M.E., The Process of Social Organisation, Holt, Rinehart and Winston, New York, 1970, especially pp.49-50 and 338.
62. This argument is developed in The Outer Circle Policy Unit, A New Perspective on the National Health Service, London, December 1978. The report was written by the author with assistance from a multi-disciplinary group (see note 40 above) and was submitted to the Royal Commission on the NHS. The main theme of the report is that structural change should succeed, rather than precede, process change and that the starting point should be the ethic of service to the patient. This involves a reversal in current thinking about organisational issues in health care where the tendency has been to focus on structure and to push to the background the complex relations between individuals which make up the real operating system. See also, Personal Social

Services Council, _Collaboration in Community Care - A Discussion Document_, HMSO, London, 1978; Towell, D. and Harries, C., _eds_., _Innovation in Patient Care_, Croom Helm, London, 1979; Weir, R.D., 'Towards a simpler organisation', _Hospital and Health Services Review_, _75_, December 1979, pp. 425-8.

63. Robinson, D. and Henry, S., _Self-Help and Health_, Martin Robertson, London, 1977, p.141.
64. See Wiseman, C., 'Selection of Major Planning Issues', _Policy Sciences_, _9_, 1978, pp.71-86; also, Brown, _op.cit_., Chapter 11.
65. See Bosanquet, _op.cit_.
66. Haywood, Stuart, 'Team management in the NHS - what is it all about?', _Health and Social Service Journal_, 5 October 1979, Centre Eight Papers, pp.B53-60.
67. Cornford, James, 'An Alternative Britain?', _Political Quarterly_, _51_, 1980, p.39.
68. Self, P., 'Nonsense on stilts - Roskill', _New Society_, 2 July 1970. The argument is developed in Hunter, David J., _Managerial Efficiency versus Political Efficiency: How this affects Accountability in the Reorganised NHS_, unpublished MA dissertation, Department of Politics, University of Edinburgh, September 1973.

Appendix I

List of Interviews *

1. Health Boards (Alpha and Beta) **

2 Chairmen
2 Vice-Chairmen
16 Members

2 Secretaries ***
2 Treasurers ***
2 Chief Administrative Medical Officers
2 Chief Area Nursing Officers
1 Chief Administrative Dental Officer
1 Chief Administrative Pharmaceutical Officer
1 Area Personnel Officer

4 District Administrators ***
3 District Finance Officers
2 District Medical Officers
2 District Nursing Officers
1 District Management Accountant
1 District Personnel Officer

3 Sector Administrators

3 Chairmen, professional advisory committees (AMC, ANMC, APC)
1 Secretary, APC

2. <u>Scottish Office/Scottish Home and Health Department</u>

1 Assistant Secretary, Scottish Office (Finance Division)
1 Secretary, SHHD
2 Undersecretaries, SHHD

3. <u>Other</u>

1 Former Principal Officer, Manpower Division, Common Services Agency
1 Former Treasurer, Grampian Health Board

* Only formal or semi-formal interviews have been listed. In addition, there were innumerable informal conversations both with those roles listed above and with others.

** Three members of Alpha declined to be interviewed because they had been newly appointed. A fourth member was absent during the interview period. Members of Beta were not interviewed for two reasons: (1) there was an access problem. The Secretary was reluctant to allow me to interview members at the time I had chosen to do so because the Secretary of State was about to announce membership changes for all boards. These changes were in fact not announced for some months; (2) it was apparent from informal discussions with a few of the members, and from other evidence, that Beta's members shared similar views to those help by members of Alpha. Nevertheless, interviews would have been conducted had it not been for the problems identified under (1) above.

*** Re-interviews were conducted with some, or all, of these roles.

Appendix II

Abbreviations

AEG	Area Executive Group
AHA	Area Health Authority
AMC	Area Medical Committee
BoM	Board of Management
BPM	Bureaucratic Politics Model
CADO	Chief Administrative Dental Officer
CAMO	Chief Administrative Medical Officer
CAPO	Chief Administrative Pharmaceutical Officer
CANO	Chief Area Nursing Officer
CHC	Community Health Council
CMS	Community Medicine Specialist
DSA	Dental Surgery Assistant
DHSS	Department of Health and Social Security
DF	Development Funds
DA	District Administrator
DDO	District Dental Officer
DEG	District Executive Group
DFO	District Finance Officer

DGH	District General Hospital
DMA	District Management Accountant
DMO	District Medical Officer
DNO	District Nursing Officer
DPO	District Personnel Officer
GP	General Practitioner
GNP	Gross National Product
HMSO	Her Majesty's Stationery Office
IHSA	Institute of Health Service Administrators
IOR	Institute for Operational Research
LHC	Local Health Council
MAS	Medical Advisory Structure
MOH	Medical Officer of Health
MD	Mentally Disordered
NHS	National Health Service
PRC	Policy and Resources Committee
PSSC	Personal Social Services Council
RAM	Rational Actor Model
RHB	Regional Hospital Board
RAWP	Resource Allocation Working Party
SED	Scottish Education Department
SHARE	Scottish Health Authorities Revenue Equalisation
SHHD	Scottish Home and Health Department
SHAS	Scottish Hospital Advisory Service
SHC	Scottish Hospital Costs
SSRC	Social Science Research Council
SOP	Standard Operating Procedure
UK	United Kingdom

Bibliography

ABEL-SMITH, B — Value for Money in Health Services, Heinemann, London, 1976.

ABRAMS, P — 'Community Care: Some Research Problems and Priorities', in Barnes, J. & Connelly, N., eds. Social Care Research, Policy Studies Institute/DHSS, London, 1978.

ADAMS, R & PREISS, J eds., — Human Organisation Research, Dorsey Press, Illinois, 1960.

ALBROW, M — Bureaucracy, Macmillan, London, 1973.

ALDEN, J & MORGAN, R — Regional Planning: A Comprehensive View, Heath & Reach, Leighton Buzzard, 1974.

ALLEN, C H — 'The Study of Scottish Politics: A Bibliographical Sermon' in Drucker, N and Drucker, H.M., eds., The Scottish Government Yearbook 1980, Paul Harris, Edinburgh, 1979.

ALLEN, D — Hospital Planning, Pitman Medical, London, 1979.

ALLISON, G T — Essence of Decision, Little, Brown & Co., Boston, 1971.

ALLISON, G T & HALPERIN, M H — 'Bureaucratic Politics', World Politics, 24, Spring 1972.

ARMSTRONG, D — 'The Decline of the Medical Hegemony: A Review of Government Reports during the NHS', Social Science and Medicine, 10, No.3/4, March/April, 1976.

ASSOCIATION OF CHIEF ADMINISTRATORS OF HEALTH AUTHORITIES — A Review of the Management of the Reorganised NHS, December 1975.

BACHRACH, P & BARATZ, M S — 'The Two Faces of Power', American Political Science Review, 56, 1962.

BACHRACH, P & BARATZ, M S — 'Decisions and Non-decisions: An Analytical Framework', American Political Science Review, 57, 1963.

BACHRACH, P & BARATZ, M S — Power and Poverty, Oxford University Press, New York, 1970.

BAKER, R J S — Administrative Theory and Public Administration, Hutchison, London, 1972.

BALL, D J — 'The Blind Men and the Elephant: a critique of bureaucratic politics theory', Australian Outlook, 28, 1974.

BARBER, J D — Power in Committees, Rand McNally & Co., Chicago, 1966.

BARNARD, C I — The Functions of the Executive, Cambridge, Massachusetts, 1966.

BARNARD, K & HAM, C — 'The Reallocation of Resources', The Lancet, 26 June 1976.

BARNARD, K & LEE, K, eds. — NHS Reorganisation: Issues and Prospects, The Nuffield Centre for Health Services Studies, University of Leeds, 1974.

BARNARD, K & LEE, K, eds. — Conflicts in the National Health Service, Croom Helm, London, 1977.

BATTISTELLA, R & CHESTER, T E — 'Reorganisation of the NHS: Background and Issues in England's Quest for a Comprehensive-Integrated Planning and Delivery System', The Milbank Memorial Fund Quarterly, 51, No.4, 1973.

BATTISTELLA, R & SMITH, D — 'Towards a Definition of Health Services Management: A Humanist Orientation', International Journal of Health Services, 4, No.4, 1974.

BAUER, R & GERGEN, K, eds. — The Study of Policy Formation, Free Press, New York, 1968.

BECKER, H et al, eds. — Institutions and the Person, Aldine Publishing Co., Chicago, 1968.

BLANDFORD, J — 'Appraising Quality and Effectiveness in Australia', in Paine, L, ed. The Health Service Administrator: Innovator or Catalyst?, King Edward's Hospital Fund for London, London, 1978.

BOADEN, N — _Urban Policy-Making_, Cambridge University Press, London, 1971.

BOCHEL, D & MACLARAN, M — _The Establishment and Development of Local Health Councils_, Scottish Health Service Studies 41, SHHD, Edinburgh, 1979.

BODDY, D — 'An Experiment in the Long-Term Planning of Health Services', _Public Administration_, _57_, Summer 1979.

BOOTH, T A, _ed_. — _Planning for Welfare_, Blackwell and Robertson, Oxford, 1979.

BOSANQUET, N & TOWNSEND, P, _eds_. — _Labour and Equality_, Heinemann, London, 1980.

BOYD, K M, _ed_. — _The Ethics of Resource Allocation in Health Care_, University of Edinburgh, Edinburgh, 1979.

BRAYBROOKE, D & LINDBLOM, C — _A Strategy of Decision_, Free Press, New York, 1963.

BRITISH HOSPITAL JOURNAL — 'Green Light for Scottish Green Paper', 11 April 1969.

BRITISH MEDICAL JOURNAL — 'Contemporary Themes: Priorities', 12 June 1976.

BROWN, M — 'Priorities for health and personal social services', in Jones, K., _ed_, _The Year Book of Social Policy in Britain 1976_, Routledge & Kegan Paul, London, 1977.

BROWN, R G S — _The Administrative Process in Britain_, Allen & Unwin, London, 1970.

BROWN, R G S — 'Reorganising the Health Service', in Jone, K., ed, The Year Book of Social Policy in Britain, 1971, Routledge & Kegan Paul, London, 1972.

BROWN, R G S, et al — Humberside Reorganisation Project - 4 reports:
1. Preparations for Change, April 1973;
2. Waiting for Guidance, November 1973;
3. The Shadow & The Substance, June 1974;
4. New Bottles: Old Wine?, September 1975, Institute for Health Studies, University of Hull.

BROWN, R G S — The Changing National Health Service, Routledge & Kegan Paul, London, 1973.

BROWN, R G S — The Management of Welfare, Fontana, London, 1975.

BROWN, R G S — 'Coming to the fork in the reorganised road', Health and Social Service Journal, 4 February 1977.

BROWN, R G S — 'Accountability and control in the National Health Service', Health and Social Service Journal, Centre Eight Papers, October 1977.

BROWN, R G S — Reorganising the National Health Service: A Case Study of Administrative Change, Blackwell/Robertson, Oxford, 1979.

BRUYN, S T — The Human Perspective in Sociology, Prentice-Hall, New Jersey, 1966.

BURLING, T, et al — The Give and Take in Hospitals, Putnam, New York, 1956.

BURNS, T & STALKER, G M — The Management of Innovation, Tavistock, London, 1961.

BUXTON, M J & KLEIN, R — 'Distribution of Hospital Provision: Policy Themes and Resource Variations', British Medical Journal, 8 February 1975.

CAMERON, D — 'Management in the NHS', in Reekie, W.D and Hunt, N.C., eds., Management in the Social and Safety Services, Tavistock, London, 1974.

CARPENTER, M — 'The New Managerialism and Professionalism in Nursing', in Stacey, M. et al, eds., Health and the Division of Labour, Croom Helm, London, 1976.

CARRIER, J & KENDALL, I — 'Social policy and social change - explanations of the development of social policy', Journal of Social Policy, 2, 3, 1973.

CASTLES, F G, et al., eds. — Decisions, Organisations and Society, second edition, Penguin, Harmondsworth, 1976.

CHAPMAN, R — Decision Making, Routledge & Kegan Paul, London, 1968.

CHESTER, T E & DONALD, B L — 'Social change and NHS reorganisation', <u>The Hospital and Health Services Review</u>, <u>72</u>, No.6, 1976.

CHESTER, T E — 'One Year Later - Impressions and Reflections', <u>The Hospital and Health Services Review</u>, <u>71</u>, 1975.

CICOUREL, A & KITSUSE, J — <u>The Educational Decision-Makers</u>, Bobbs-Merrill, New York, 1963.

CLARKE, M G — 'Great Britain: The Quest for Efficiency', in Cornford, J.P., <u>ed</u>., <u>The Failure of the State</u>, Croom Helm, London, 1975.

COCHRANE, A L — <u>Effectiveness and Efficiency: Random Reflections on Health Services</u>, Nuffield Provincial Hospitals Trust, London, 1972.

COOPER, M H — 'Rationing health', <u>New Society</u>, 18 April 1974.

COOPER, M H — 'Rationing and Financing Health Care Resources', in Reekie, W.D. and Hunt, N.C., <u>eds</u>., <u>Management in the Social and Safety Services</u>, Tavistock, London, 1974.

COOPER, M H — <u>Rationing Health Care</u>, Croom Helm, London, 1975.

CORNFORD, J P — 'Review Article: The Illusion of Decision', <u>British Journal of Political Science</u>, <u>4</u>, 1974.

CORNFORD, J P — 'An Alternative Britain?', <u>Political Quarterly</u>, <u>51</u>, 1980.

CRECINE, J P — Governmental Problem-Solving, Rand McNally and Co., Chicago, 1969.

CROSSMAN, R H S — A Politician's View of Health Service Planning, University of Glasgow, 1972.

CULYER, A J — 'Health: the social cost of doctors' discretion', New Society, 27 February 1975.

CULYER, A J — Need and the NHS: Economics and Social Choice, Martin Robertson, London, 1976.

DANZIGER, J N — 'Assessing Incrementalism in British Municipal Budgeting', British Journal of Political Science, 6, 1976.

DANZIGER, J N — 'A Comment on "The Politics of the Budgetary Process in English Local Government"', Political Studies, 26, No.1, 1978.

DANZIGER, J N — Making Budgets: Public Resource Allocation, Sage, London, 1979.

DAVIES, C — 'Professionals in Organisations: Some Preliminary Observations on Hospital Consultants', Sociological Review, 20, 1972.

DAVIES, C — 'Hospital Consultants and Collective Action', amended draft of a paper presented to the BSA Medical Sociology Conference, York, November 1973, unpublished.

DAVIS, A G — 'An Unequivocal Change of Policy: Prevention Health and Medical Sociology', Social Science and Medicine, 13A, March 1978.

DEARLOVE, J — The Politics of Policy in Local Government, Cambridge University Press, Cambridge, 1973.

DIMMOCK, S & BARNARD, K — 'Relationships and Communications', in Raybould, E, ed. A Guide for Nurse Managers, Blackwell, Oxford, 1977.

DINGWALL, R — 'The End of Medical Dominance?' Health and Social Service Journal, 4 January 1975.

DONALD, B L — 'Volunteers Retained as Managers: NHS Reorganisation Changes Authority Members' Role', Public Administration, 54, Autumn 1975.

DONNISON, D, et al — Social Policy and Administration Revisited, Allen & Unwin, London, 1975.

DRAPER, P & SMART, A — The Future of our Health Care, Guy's Hospital Medical School, London, 1972.

DRAPER, P & SMART, A — 'Social Service and Health Policy in the UK: Some Contributions of the Social Sciences to the Bureaucratisation of the NHS', International Journal of Health Services, 4, 1974.

DRAPER, P, _et al_ — 'The Organisation of Health Care: A Critical View of the 1974 Reorganisation of the NHS', in Tuckett, D, _ed._, _An Introduction to Medical Sociology_, Tavistock, London, 1976.

DROR, Y — 'Muddling Through - "Science" or Inertia?', _Public Administration Review_, _24_, September 1964.

DROR, Y — _Public Policy-Making Re-examined_, Leonard Hill Books, Aylesbury, 1973.

DUBIN, R — 'Stability of Human Organisation', in Haire, M, _ed._, _Modern Organisation Theory_, Wiley & Sons, Chicago, 1959.

ECKSTEIN, H — _The English Health Service_, Harvard University Press, Massachusetts, 1964.

EDWARDS III, G C & SHARKANSKY, I — _The Policy Predicament_, Freeman & Co., San Francisco, 1978.

ETZIONI, A — _Modern Organizations_, Prentice-Hall, New Jersey, 1964.

FARNDALE, J, _ed._ — _Trends in the National Health Service_, Pergamon Press, Oxford, 1964.

FOOT, M — _Aneurin Bevan 1945-60_, _Vol.2_, Paladin, London, 1973.

FORSYTH, G — _Doctors and State Medicine_, Pitman Medical, London, 1966.

FREIDSON, E, _ed_. _The Hospital in Modern Society_, Free Press, New York, 1963.

FREIDSON, E _Professional Dominance_, Atherton Press, New York, 1970.

FREIDSON, E _Profession of Medicine_, Dodd, Mead & Co., New York, 1970.

FREIDSON, E, _ed_. _The Professions and their Prospects_, Sage, Beverly Hills, 1973.

FRIEND, J K & JESSOP, W N _Local Government and Strategic Choice_, second edition, Pergamon Press, Oxford, 1977.

FRIEND, J K, _et al_ _Public Planning: the inter-corporate dimension_, Tavistock, London, 1974.

FRIEND, J K 'Inter-Organisational Decision-Making in the Provision of Local Community Services: A Framework for the Selection of Research Priorities', IOR/876, Institute for Operational Research, London, October 1975.

GARRETT, J _The Management of Government_, Penguin, Harmondsworth, 1972.

GARRETT, R D _Hospitals: a systems approach_, Auerbach, Philadelphia, 1973.

GENTLE, P H & FORSYTHE, J M 'Revenue Allocation in the Reorganised NHS', _British Medical Journal_, 9 August 1975.

GLENNERSTER, H _Social Service Budgets and Social Policy_, Allen & Unwin, London, 1975.

GODBER, Sir G — 'Regional Devolution and the NHS', in Craven, E, ed., Regional Devolution and Social Policy, Centre for Studies in Social Policy/Macmillan, London, 1975.

GODBER, Sir G — The Health Service: Past, Present and Future, Heath Clark Lectures, University of London, 1975.

GODBER, Sir G — Attainable Goals in Health, The 16th Maurice Bloch Lecture, Glasgow University Press, Glasgow, 1976.

GOLD, R L — 'Roles in sociological field observation', Social Forces, 36, 1958.

GORE, W J — Administrative Decision-Making: a heuristic model, Wiley & Sons, New York, 1964.

GORTNER, H F — Administration in the Public Sector, Wiley & Sons, New York, 1977.

GOULDNER, A W — Patterns of Industrial Bureaucracy, Free Press, New York, 1964.

GOURLAY, R — 'Team and Consensus Management: Horse or Camel?', in Barnard, K and Lee, K, eds., NHS Reorganisation: Issues and Prospects, op.cit.

GREEN, S — The Hospital: an organisational analysis, Blackie, Glasgow, 1974.

GREEN, S — 'Professional/Bureaucratic Conflict: The Case of the Medical Profession in the National Health Service', Sociological Review, 23, 1975.

GREENWOOD, R et al — 'The Politics of the Budgetary Process in English Local Government', Political Studies, 25, No.1, 1977.

GREENWOOD, R et al — 'A Rejoinder to Danziger's Comment', Political Studies, 26, No.1, 1978.

GREENWOOD, R — 'The Local Authority Budgetary Process' in Booth, op.cit.

HAH, CHONG-DO & LINDQUIST, R — 'The '52 Steel Seizure Revisited: A Systematic Study in Presidential Decision-Making, Administrative Science Quarterly, 20, December 1975.

HALL, P et al — Change, Choice and Conflict in Social Policy, Heinemann, London, 1975.

HALL, R H — Organisations: Structure and Process, 2nd edition, Prentice-Hall, New Jersey, 1977.

HALLAS, J — CHCs in Action, Nuffield Provincial Hospitals Trust, London, 1976.

HAMILTON, D — 'Fair SHARE', The Scotsman, 31 August 1977.

HAYWOOD, S C — Managing the Health Service, Allen & Unwin, London, 1974.

HAYWOOD, S C — 'The tug of war between local and national needs', Health and Social Service Journal, 28 August 1976.

HAYWOOD, S C — Decision Making in the NHS: Consensus or Constipation?, King's Fund Project Paper, London, 1977.

HAYWOOD, S C — 'More democracy for the NHS?', The Hospital & Health Services Review, 73, No.4, April 1977.

HAYWOOD, S C — 'Team management in the NHS - what is it all about?', Health and Social Service Journal, Centre Eight Papers, 5 October 1979.

HAYWOOD, S C et al — 'The Outcome of NHS Re-organisation: Structural Change and Implementation of Social Policy', Public Administration Bulletin, No.31, December 1979.

HAYWOOD, S C & ALASZEWSKI, A — The NHS - Who Rules?, Croom Helm, London, forthcoming.

HECLO, H — 'The Councillor's Job', Public Administration, 47, 1969.

HECLO, H — 'Review Article: Policy Analysis', British Journal of Political Science, 2, 1972.

HECLO, H & WILDAVSKY, A — The Private Government of Public Money, Macmillan, London, 1974.

HECLO, H — Modern Social Politics in Britain and Sweden, Yale University Press, London, 1975.

HECLO, H — 'Social Politics and Policy Impacts', in Holden Jr, M and Dresang, D.L. eds., What Government Does, Sage, Beverly Hills, 1975.

HEIDENHEIMER, A J et al — Comparative Public Policy, Macmillan, London, 1976.

HELLER, T — Restructuring the Health Service, Croom Helm, London, 1978.

HIGGINS, J — The Poverty Business: Britain and America, Blackwell & Robertson, Oxford, 1978.

HILL, M J — The Sociology of Public Administration, Weidenfeld & Nicolson, London, 1972.

HOARE, J — 'Bread and Games', Hospital and Health Services Review, 75, October 1979.

HOOD, C C — The Limits of Administration, Wiley & Sons, London, 1976.

THE HOSPITAL & HEALTH SERVICES REVIEW — 'Editorial', 67, No.9, September 1971.

THE HOSPITAL & HEALTH SERVICES REVIEW — 'Scottish objectives', 69, No.7, July 1973.

THE HOSPITAL & HEALTH SERVICES REVIEW — 'Priorities', 72, No.5, May 1976.

HOUSE OF COMMONS — *Health Services Bill No.98*, HMSO, London 1979.

HOWICK, C — 'Budgeting and Corporate Planning in Cheshire', *CES Review*, May 1978.

HUNTER, D J — 'Managerial Efficiency v. Political Efficience: how this affects accountability in the reorganised NHS', MA dissertation, Department of Politics, University of Edinburgh, September 1973, unpublished.

HUNTER, D J — 'The Application of Economic Analysis in the Running of the National Health Service', MA dissertation, Department of Politics, University of Edinburgh, April 1974, unpublished.

HUNTER, D J — *Decisions and Resources in the National Health Service in Scotland*, Ph.D. thesis, University of Edinburgh, 1979.

HUNTER, D J — 'Coping with uncertainty: decisions and resources within health authorities', *Sociology of Health and Illness*, *1*, June 1979.

HUNTER, D J — 'Patterns of Organisation for Health: A Systems Overview of the National Health Service in the United Kingdom', unpublished paper presented to SSRC Workshop on the Comparative Study of the Social Services in the UK, Edinburgh, September 1979.

HUNTER, D J	'Decision-Making in Health Authorities: Research Findings and Policy Implications', *Research Bulletin*, Department of Social Administration, University of Edinburgh, Number 3, October 1979.
HUNTER, D J	'Practice: decisions and resources in the National Health Service (Scotland)' in Boyd, *op.cit*.
HUNTER, T D	'Arena or Amoeba: Managing the Health Network', *The Hospital and Health Services Review, 67*, 1971.
HUNTER, T D	'Scots Wha Hae', *Health and Social Service Journal*, 7 July 1973.
HUNTER, D	'The reorganised Health Service: a Scottish Perspective', in Clarke, M.G. and Drucker, H.M. *eds*., *Our Changing Scotland: a Yearbook of Scottish Government 1976-77*, EUSPB, Edinburgh, 1976.
ILLICH, I	*Limits to Medicine*, Penguin, Harmondsworth, 1977.
ILLICH, I *et al*	*Disabling Professions*, Marion Boyars, London, 1977.
ILLSLEY, R	'Promotion to observer status', *Social Science & Medicine*, *9*, 1975.

INSTITUTE OF HEALTH SERVICE ADMINISTRATORS (IHSA) — The Role of Unit and Sector Administrators in the National Health Service, report of a joint working party, IHSA, London, 1976.

INSTITUTE FOR OPERATIONAL RESEARCH (IOR) — Programme of Studies in Health Planning April 1974 - May 1976, IOR/883R, Edinburgh, May 1976.

JAQUES, E ed, — Health Services, Heinemann, London, 1978.

JOHNSON, T J — Professions and Power, Macmillan, London, 1972.

JUDGE, K — Rationing Social Services, Heinemann, London, 1978.

KAUFMAN, H — 'The next step in case studies', Public Administration Review, 18, 1958.

KEELING, D — Management in Government, Allen & Unwin, London, 1972.

KELLAS, J G — The Scottish Political System, second edition, Cambridge University Press, London, 1975.

KEMPNER, A T & WILLS, G eds. — Management Thinkers, Penguin, Harmondsworth, 1978.

KLEIN, R — 'Mismanaging the NHS', Management Today, December 1971.

KLEIN, R — 'Accountability in the NHS', Political Quarterly, 42, 1971.

KLEIN, R — 'An Anatomy of the NHS', New Society, 28 June 1973.

KLEIN, R — 'NHS: After Reorganisation', Political Quarterly, 44, 1973.

KLEIN, R — 'Policy Making in the National Health Service', Political Studies, 22, March 1974.

KLEIN, R — 'Policy problems and policy perceptions in the National Health Service', Policy and Politics, 2, No.3, 1974.

KLEIN, R ed. — Social Policy and Public Expenditure 1975: Inflation and Priorities, Centre for Studies in Social Policy, London, 1975.

KLEIN, R — 'Notes and Comments: A Reply', British Journal of Political Science, 6, 1976.

KLEIN, R — 'Reorganisation: what went wrong', New Society, 22 September 1977.

KOGAN, M — The Politics of Education, Penguin, Harmondsworth, 1971.

KOGAN, M — County Hall: The Role of the Chief Education Officer, Penguin, Harmondsworth, 1974.

KOGAN, M — Educational Policy-Making, Allen & Unwin, London, 1975.

KOGAN, M — 'Book review', Political Quarterly, 47, 1976.

KOGAN, M — 'Notes and Comments', British Journal of Political Science, 6, 1976.

KOVNER, A R — 'Hospital Board Members as Policy-Makers: Role, Priorities and Qualifications', Medical Care, 12, December 1974.

LALONDE, M — A New Perspective on the Health of Canadians, Ministry of National Health & Welfare, Canada, April 1974.

LA PORTE, ed. — Organised Social Complexity: Challenge to Politics and Policy, Princeton University Press, New Jersey, 1975.

LEE, J M & WOOD, B — The Scope of Local Initiative: a study of Cheshire county council 1961-74, Martin Robertson, London, 1974.

LEE, K — 'Public Expenditure, Planning and Local Democracy', in Barnard, K and Lee, K eds. Conflicts in the National Health Service, op.cit.

LEE, K & MILLS, A — 'The contribution of economics to health service planning', Health & Social Service Journal, Centre Eight Papers, 8 February 1979.

LEVIN, P H — 'On Decisions and Decision-Making', Public Administration, 50, Spring 1972.

LEVITT, R — The Reorganised National Health Service, Croom Helm, London, 1976.

LEWIS, J & WEINER, S — 'Reorganisation: The First Year', _British Medical Journal_, 5 July 1975.

LIND, G & WISEMAN, C — 'Setting Health Priorities: A Review of Concepts and Approaches', _Journal of Social Policy_, _7_, 4, 1978.

LINDBLOM, C — 'The Science of "Muddling Through"', _Public Administration Review_, _19_, 1959.

LINDBLOM, C — 'Contexts for Change and Strategy: a Reply', _Public Administration Review_, _24_, 1964.

LINDBLOM, C — _The Policy-Making Process_, Prentice-Hall, New Jersey, 1968.

LINDSEY, A — _Socialised Medicine in England and Wales_, Oxford University Press, London, 1962.

LOGAN, R F L _et al_ — _Dynamics of Medical Care_, London School of Hygiene & Tropical Medicine, 1972.

LOWI, T — 'Decision-Making vs. Policy-Making: towards an antidote for technocracy', _Public Administration Review_, _30_, No.3, May/June 1970.

LUCKMAN, T _ed_. — _Phenomenology and Sociology_, Penguin, Harmondsworth, 1978.

LUKES, S — _Power_, Macmillan, London, 1974.

MACKENZIE, W J M — *Power and Responsibility in Health Care*,. Oxford University Press for Nuffield Provincial Hospitals Trust, London, 1979.

McGLEW, T & ROBERTSON, A — 'Social Change and the Shifting Boundaries of Discretion in Medicine', unpublished paper presented to SSRC Workshop on Discretion, Cambridge, July 1979.

McKEOWN, T — *The Role of Medicine: Dream, Mirage or Nemesis*, Nuffield Provincial Hospitals Trust, London, 1976.

McKINSEY & CO — *Health Care: The Growing Dilemma*, New York, 1974.

McKINSEY & CO — *Realizing the Promise of a National Health Service*; submission by J Banham *et al* to the Royal Commission on the NHS, London, January 1977.

MADDOX, G L — 'Muddling Through: Planning for Health Care in England', *Medical Care*, *9*, No.5, September-October 1971.

MADGE, J — *The Tools of Social Science*, Tavistock, London, 1953.

MANN, P H — *Methods of Sociological Enquiry*, Blackwell, London, 1971.

MANSON, T — 'Management, the Professions and the Unions: A Social Analysis of Change in the National Health Service', in Stacey, M *et al*, *eds. Health & the Division of Labour*, Croom Helm, London, 1976.

MANT, A — _The Rise and Fall of the British Manager_, Macmillan, London, 1977.

MARCH, J G & SIMON, H — _Organisations_, Wiley & Sons, New York, 1958.

MARMOR, T — _The Politics of Medicare_, Routledge & Kegan Paul, London, 1970.

MARTIN, M — _Colleagues or Competitors?_, Occasional Papers on Social Administration No.31, Bell, London, 1969.

MAXWELL, R — 'Anomie in the NHS - A McKinsey View', _British Medical Journal_, 16 August 1975.

MAXWELL, R — 'Management arrangements - sense or nonsense?', _The Hospital & Health Services Review_, _72_, No.3, 1976.

MAXWELL, R — 'An Introduction', in Paine, L. _ed_. _The Health Service Administrator: Innovator or Catalyst?_, King Edward's Hospital Fund for London, London, 1978.

MECHANIC, D — _Public Expectations and Health Care_, Wiley & Sons, New York, 1972.

MEYERSON, M & BANFIELD, E C — _Politics, Planning, and the Public Process_, Free Press, New York, 1955.

MILLS, A & REYNOLDS, J — 'Centre-periphery: Can Guide-lines Bridge the Gap?', The Hospital & Health Services Review, 73, No.2, 1977.

MINTZBERG, H et al — 'The Structure of "Unstructured" Decision Processes', Administrative Science Quarterly, 21, No.2, June 1976.

MITCHELL, R — 'The first year of the re-organised Scottish Health Service', The Hospital & Health Services Review, 71, No.5, 1975.

MITCHELL, R — 'Resources in Scottish Health Services', in Paine, L. ed. The Health Service Administrator: Innovator or Catalyst?, Kind Edward's Hospital Fund for London, London, 1978.

MOONEY, G — 'Programme budgeting in an area health board', The Hospital & Health Services Review, 73, No.11, November 1977.

MORRIS, J N — 'Tomorrow's Community Physician', in Gatherer, A & Warren, M.D. eds. Management & the Health Services, P Pergamon Press, Oxford, 1971.

NELSON, R R — 'Intellectualizing about the Moon-Ghetto Metaphor: A Study of the Current Malaise of Rational Analysis of Social Problems', Policy Sciences, 5, 1974.

NEW SOCIETY 'Guide to the new NHS', 28 February 1974.

NOYCE, J *et al* 'Regional Variations in the Allocation of Financial Resources to the Community Health Services', *The Lancet*, 30 March 1974.

OFFICE OF HEALTH ECONOMICS *The NHS Reorganisation*, London, 1974.

OFFICE OF HEALTH ECONOMICS *The health care dilemma*, London, 1975.

OFFICE OF HEALTH ECONOMICS *The NHS Reorganisation*, London, 1977.

OFFICE OF HEALTH ECONOMICS *The Cost of the NHS*, Briefing No.7, October 1978.

OFFICE OF HEALTH ECONOMICS *Compendium of Health Statistics*, 3rd edition, London, 1979.

OLSEN, M E *The Process of Social Organisation*, Holt, Rinehart & Winston, New York, 1970.

THE OPEN UNIVERSITY *Health*, Course Textbook, Open University Press, 1972.

THE OUTER CIRCLE POLICY UNIT *A New Perspective on the National Health Service*, London, December, 1978.

OWEN, D *A Unified Health Service*, Pergamon Press, Oxford, 1968.

OWEN, D *In Sickness and In Health: The Politics of Medicine*, Quartet, London, 1976.

PARRY, G & MORRISS, P — 'When is a Decision not a Decision?', in Crewe, I. ed. British Political Sociology Yearbook, Vol.1, Croom Helm, London, 1974.

PETHYBRIDGE, F — 'Multi-disciplinary management and decision-making in the reorganised NHS', The Hospital & Health Services Review, 72, No.3, March 1976.

POWELL, E — Medicine and Politics, Pitman Medical, London, 1967.

POWER, J — 'Organisational Technology and Public Planning', Public Administration Australia, 30, 1971.

POWLES, J — 'On the limitations of modern medicine', Science, Medicine & Man, 1, 1973.

PRESSMAN, J L & WILDAVSKY, A — Implementation, University of California Press, Berkeley, 1973.

RADICAL STATISTICS HEALTH GROUP — Whose Priorities?, Pamphlet 1, London, 1976.

RADICAL STATISTICS HEALTH GROUP — In Defence of the NHS, London, 1977.

RAKOFF, S H & SCHAEFER, G F — 'Politics, Policy and Political Science: Theoretical Alternatives', Politics and Society, 1, No.1, 1970.

REIN, M — Social Science and Public Policy, Penguin, Harmondsworth, 1976.

RHODES, R A W — 'Centre-Local Relations', in Appendix 6: The Relationship between Central & Local Government: Evidence & Commissioned Work, Report of the Committee of Inquiry into Local Government Finance (Layfield), Cmnd.6543, HMSO, London, 1976.

RHODES, R A W — 'Research into Central-Local Relations in Britain: A Framework for Analysis' in SSRC, Central-Local Government Relationships, London, 1979.

RIBBINS, P M & BROWN, R J — 'Policy Making in English Local Government: The Case of Secondary School Reorganisation', Public Administration, 57, Summer 1979.

RICKARD, J H — 'Per capita expenditure of the English area health authorities', British Medical Journal, 31 January 1976.

RIDLEY, F F — 'Public Administration: Cause for Discontent', Public Administration, 50, Spring 1972.

RIVLIN, A — 'Obstacles to Social Progress: Why Can't We Get Things Done', Washington Post, 22 July 1971.

ROBINSON, D & HENRY, S — Self-help and Health, Martin Robertson, London, 1977.

ROBSON, J — 'The NHS and Co. Inc.?', International Journal of Health Services, 3, 1973.

ROSS, J S — *The National Health Service in Great Britain*, Oxford University Press, London, 1952.

ROWBOTTOM, R *et al* — *Hospital Organisation*, Heinemann, London, 1973.

RUGGIE, J G — 'Complexity, Planning and Public Order', in La Porte, *op.cit*.

RYAN, M — 'The Tripartite Administrative Structure of the NHS - its Genesis and Reform', *Social & Economic Administration*, *6*, 1972.

RYAN, M — 'The Royal Commission on the NHS - Origins and Prospect', *Social & Economic Administration*, *11*, No.3, Autumn 1977.

SAVAGE, G — 'The executive group: a secretary's view', *The Hospital & Health Services Review*, *72*, No.6, 1976.

SCHATZMAN, L & STRAUSS, A — *Field Research*, Prentice-Hall, New Jersey, 1973.

SCHON, D — *Beyond the Stable State*, Penguin, Harmondsworth, 1973.

SCHULTZE, C — *The Politics and Economics of Public Spending*, The Brookings Institution, Washington, 1968.

SELF, P — 'Nonsense on stilts - Roskill', *New Society*, 2 July 1970.

SELF P — 'Is Comprehensive Planning Possible and Rational?', *Policy & Politics*, *2*, No.3, 1974.

SELF, P — Administrative Theories and Politics, second edition, Allen & Unwin, London, 1977.

SHARKANSKY, I — The Routines of Politics, Van Nostrand Reinhold, New York, 1970.

SIMON, H A — Administrative Behaviour, Free Press, New York, 1957.

SMITH, A — 'Are we any healthier?', New Society, 8 September 1977.

SMITH, B — Policy Making in British Government: An Analysis of Power and Rationality, Martin Robertson, London, 1976.

SOCIAL SCIENCE RESEARCH COUNCIL — Health and Health Policy: priorities for research, report of an advisory panel to the Research Initiatives Board, London, June 1977.

SPENCER, J A — Management in Hospitals, Faber, London, 1967.

STACEY, F — British Government 1966-1975: Years of Reform, Oxford University Press, London, 1975.

STANYER, J — Understanding Local Government, Fontana, London, 1976.

STANYER, J & SMITH, B — Administering Health, Fontana, London, 1976.

STEELE, R & MOONEY, G — 'SHARE: the case for equity in health', The Scotsman, 13 September 1977.

STEIN, H *ed.* — *Public Administration and Policy Development*, Harcourt, Brace & World, New York, 1952.

STEVENS, R — *Medical Practice in Modern Britain*, Yale University Press, New York, 1966.

STEWART, J D — 'The NHS - the structural problem', *The Hospital & Health Services Review*, *73*, No.9, September 1977.

STRAUSS, A *et al* — *Psychiatric Ideologies and Institutions*, Free Press, New York, 1964.

THE SUNDAY TIMES — 'Crisis in the NHS?', 16 July 1978; 23 July 1978; 30 July 1978.

SUNDERLAND, J C — 'Health Administration and the Jaundice of Reorganisation', in Barnard, K and Lee, K. *eds*. *Conflicts in the National Health Service*, *op.cit*.

SUSSER, M W & WATSON, W — *Sociology in Medicine*, Oxford University Press, London, 1971.

TAYLOR, R — 'The local health system: an ethnography of interest-groups and decision-making', *Social Science & Medicine*, *11*, 1977.

TEELING-SMITH, G — 'Cost-benefit paralysis', *Nursing Times*, 22 January 1976.

TEELING-SMITH, G — 'Counting the cost of growth', *Health & Social Service Journal*, 14 August 1976.

THOMSON, W — 'The executive group: a CAMO's view', The Hospital & Health Services Review, 72, No.6, 1976.

TOWELL, D — 'Making Reorganisation Work: Challenges and Dilemmas in the Development of Community Medicine', in Barnard, K & Lee, K. eds. Conflicts in the National Health Service, op.cit.

TOWELL, D & HARRIES, C eds. — Innovation in Patient Care, Croom Helm, London, 1979.

TOWNSEND, P — 'Inequality and the Health Service', The Lancet, 15 June 1974.

TUCKETT, D ed. — An Introduction to Medical Sociology, Tavistock, London, 1976.

UNIT FOR THE STUDY OF HEALTH POLICY — Re-thinking Community Medicine: Towards a Renaissance in Public Health?, Department of Community Medicine, Guy's Hospital Medical School, London, June 1979.

WATKIN, B — 'Health care planning - comprehensive planning', Health & Social Service Journal, 20 September 1975.

WATKIN, B — 'Health care planning - participation', Health & Social Service Journal, 27 September 1975.

WATKIN, B — The National Health Service: The First Phase 1948-1974 and After, Allen & Unwin, London, 1978.

WEBB, A — 'Power and Policy Making', Social & Economic Administration, 11, No.3, Autumn 1977.

WEIR, R D — 'Towards a simpler organisation', Hospital and Health Services Review, 75, December 1979.

WILDAVSKY, A — The Politics of the Budgetary Process, Little, Brown & Co. Boston, 1964.

WILDAVSKY, A — 'Doing Better and Feeling Worse: The Political Pathology of Health Policy', in Knowles, J H ed. Doing Better and Feeling Worse, Norton & Co. New York, 1977.

WILLCOCKS, A J — The Creation of the National Health Service, Routledge & Kegan Paul, London, 1967.

WISEMAN, C — 'Selection of Major Planning Issues', Policy Sciences, 9, 1978.

WISEMAN, C — 'Strategic Planning in the Scottish NHS - A Mixed-Scanning Approach', Long Range Planning, April 1979.

WISEMAN, C — 'Policy-Making for the Scottish Health Services at National Level', in Drucker, N and Drucker, H M eds., The Scottish Government Yearbook 1980, Paul Harris, Edinburgh, 1979.

YOUNG, K — '"Values" in the Policy Process', Policy and Politics, 5, 1977.

Official Documents and Reports

Department of Health & Social Security (DHSS) — NHS 20th Anniversary Conference Report, HMSO, London, 1968.

DHSS — The Future Structure of the National Health Service, HMSO, London, 1970.

DHSS — National Health Service Reorganisation: Consultative Document, London, 1971.

DHSS — Management Arrangements for the Reorganised National Health Service, HMSO, London, 1972.

DHSS — National Health Service Reorganisation - England, Cmnd.5055, HMSO, London, 1972.

DHSS — Guide to Planning in the National Health Service, HMSO, London, 1975.

DHSS — Decisions and Resources, HMSO, London, 1976.

DHSS — The NHS planning system, London, June 1976.

DHSS — Sharing Resources for Health in England: report of the Resource Allocation Working Party, HMSO, London, 1976.

DHSS — Prevention and Health: everybody's business, HMSO, London, 1976.

DHSS — Priorities for Health and Personal Social Services in England: A Consultative Document, HMSO, London, 1976.

DHSS — Making Whitley Work: a review of the operation of the NHS Whitley Council System (McCarthy), London, 1976.

DHSS — Priorities in the Health and Social Services: The Way Forward, HMSO, London, 1977.

DHSS — Annual Report 1976, Cmnd.6931, HMSO, London, 1977.

DHSS — National Health Service: The first thirty years (Abel-Smith, B), HMSO, London, 1978.

DHSS — Patients First, HMSO, London, 1979.

DHSS (Northern Ireland) — Consultative Paper on the Structure and Management of Health and Personal Social Services in Northern Ireland, HMSO, Belfast, 1979.

Management of Local Government (Maud) — Report, HMSO, London, 1967.

Ministry of Health/ Department of Health for Scotland — A National Health Service, Cmd.6502, HMSO, London, 1944.

Ministry of Health	The Cost of the National Health Service (Guillebaud), Cmd.9663, HMSO, London, 1956.
Ministry of Health/ SHHD	Report of the Committee on Senior Nursing Staff (Salmon), HMSO, London, 1966.
Ministry of Health	Administrative Structure of the Medical and Related Services in England and Wales, HMSO, London, 1968.
NHS Circular 1975 (GEN) 54	'Management below district level'.
NHS Circular No.1976 (GEN) 16	'Use of resources in the national health service'.
National Health Service (Scotland) Act 1978 *	HMSO, London, 1978.
National Health Service Act 1978 *	HMSO, London, 1978.
Personal Social Services Council/ Central Health Services Council/ DHSS	Collaboration in Community Care - a Discussion Document, HMSO, London, 1978.
Royal College of Physicians	A Review of the Medical Services in Great Britain (Porritt), London, 1962.
Royal Commission on the National Health Service	The Task of the Commission, HMSO, London, 1976.
Royal Commission on the National Health Service	The Working of the National Health Service (Kogan, M et al), Research Paper Number 1, HMSO, London, 1978.

---

* These Acts are consolidations of the provision of the NHS Acts 1947 to 1976.

Royal Commission on the National Health Service — *Management of Financial Resources in the National Health Service*, Research Paper Number 2, HMSO, London, 1978.

Royal Commission on the National Health Service — *Allocating health resources: A commentary on the Report of the Resource Allocation* W *Working Party* (Buxton, M J & Klein, R E), Research Paper Number 3, HMSO, London, 1978.

Royal Commission on the National Health Service — *Report*, Cmnd.7615, HMSO, London, July 1979.

Scottish Health Service Centre — *Current developments in health planning*, proceedings of conference, Edinburgh, 27 June 1975.

Scottish Health Service Centre — *Health service economics*, proceedings of conference, Edinburgh, 26 February 1976.

Scottish Health Service Planning Council — *Progress Report* by working party on health priorities, February 1977.

SHHD/Scottish Health Services Council — *Administrative Practice of Hospital Boards in Scotland* (Farquharson-Lang), HMSO, Edinburgh, 1966.

SHHD — *Organisation of Medical Work in the Hospital Service in Scotland* (Brotherston), HMSO, Edinburgh, 1967.

SHHD — *Administrative Reorganisation of the Scottish Health Services*, HMSO, Edinburgh, 1968.

SHHD — *Doctors in an Integrated Health Service*, HMSO, Edinburgh, 1971.

SHHD — Reorganisation of the Scottish Health Services, Cmnd.4734, HMSO, London, 1971.

SHHD — Health Service Reorganisation Scotland (Blue Band Circulars), HSR(72)C1 - HSR(74)C12, Edinburgh, 1972-1974.

SHHD — The Organisation of a Medical Advisory Structure, HMSO, Edinburgh, 1973.

SHHD — The National Health Service and the Community in Scotland, HMSO, Edinburgh, 1974.

SHHD — Health Services in Scotland: Report for 1974, Cmnd.6052, HMSO, Edinburgh, 1975.

SHHD — Scottish Health Service Planning Council, Report for 1974, HMSO, Edinburgh, 1975.

SHHD — Health Services in Scotland: Report for 1975, Cmnd.6506, HMSO, Edinburgh, 1976.

SHHD — The Health Service in Scotland: The Way Ahead, HMSO, Edinburgh, 1976.

SHHD — Health Services in Scotland: Report for 1976, Cmnd.6812, HMSO, Edinburgh, 1977.

SHHD — Scottish Health Service Planning Council, Report for 1976, HMSO, Edinburgh, 1977.

SHHD — Scottish Health Authorities Revenue Equalisation (SHARE): report of the Working Party on Revenue Resource Allocation, HMSO, Edinburgh, 1977.

SHHD — <u>Interim Report</u> of Working Party on Revenue Resource Allocation, September 1976; Appendix 2 of <u>SHARE</u> report.

SHHD — <u>The Medical Advisory Structure Within Health Boards in Scotland: A Review</u>, April 1977.

SHHD — Working Party on Relationships Between Health Boards and Local Authorities (Mitchell) - <u>Report</u>, HMSO, Edinburgh, 1977.

SHHD — <u>Health Services in Scotland: Report for 1977</u>, Cmnd.7237, HMSO, Edinburgh, 1978.

SHHD — Scottish Health Service Planning Council, <u>Report for 1977</u>, HMSO, Edinburgh, 1978.

SHHD — <u>The National Health Service in Scotland 1948-1978</u>, HMSO, Edinburgh, 1978.

SHHD — <u>Health Services in Scotland: Report for 1978</u>, Cmnd.7607, HMSO, Edinburgh, 1979.

SHHD/SED — <u>A Better Life: report on services for the mentally handicapped in Scotland</u>, HMSO, Edinburgh, 1979.

SHHD — <u>Structure and Management of the NHS in Scotland</u>, HMSO, Edinburgh, 1979.

Index